Vocal Fold Scar

Vocal Fold Scar

Current Concepts and Management

Edited by

Jaime Eaglin Moore, M.D., Mary J. Hawkshaw, BSN, RN, CORLN, and
Robert T. Sataloff, M.D., D.M.A., F.A.C.S.

compton
PUBLISHING

ISBN 978-1-909082-25-0

A catalogue record for this book is available from the British Library.

Cover design: David Siddall, http://www.davidsiddall.com
Cover images courtesy of Julian McGlashan, FRCS

Set in 11pt Adobe Caslon Pro by Regent Typesetting

1   2016

Contents

Contributors

Farhad Chowdhury, M.D., ENT and Allergy Associates, Voice and Swallowing Division Woodbridge, NJ., and Clinical Assistant Professor, Department of Otolaryngology – Head and Neck Surgery; Drexel University, College of Medicine, Philadelphia, PA.

Ramon A. Franco Jr, M.D., Associate Professor, Department of Otology and Laryngology, Massachusetts Eye and Ear Infirmary, Boston, MA.

Scott Hardison, M.D., Department of Otolaryngology, Virginia Commonwealth University, Richmond, VA.

Mary Hawkshaw, RN, BSN, CORLN, Research Professor, Department of Otolaryngology – Head and Neck Surgery, Drexel University College of Medicine, Philadelphia, PA.

Hayley Herbert, F.R.A.C.S., MB.ChB, Otolaryngology Fellow, Royal National Throat, Nose and Ear Hospital, London.

Shigeru Hirano, M.D., Ph.D., Department of Otolaryngology, Graduate School of Medicine, Kyoto University, Japan.

Inna Husain, M.D., Assistant Professor, Dept. of Otorhinolaryngology, Head and Neck Surgery; Director, Program for Voice, Airway, and Swallowing Disorders, Rush University Medical Center, Chicago, Il.

Aaron J. Jaworek, M.D., Laryngology Fellow, Instructor, Department of Otolaryngology – Head and Neck Surgery, Drexel University, College of Medicine, Philadelphia, PA

William E. Karle, M.D. Resident, Department of Otolaryngology – Head and Neck Surgery, New York Eye and Ear Infirmary of Mount Sinai, New York, NY.

Jaime Eaglin Moore, M.D., Assistant Professor Otolaryngology – Head and Neck Surgery, and Virginia Commonwealth University, Richmond, VA.

Michael J. Pitman, M.D., Associate Professor, Department of Otolaryngology/ Head & Neck Surgery, College of Physicians and Surgeons of Columbia University, New York, NY.

Joel E. Portnoy, M.D., Assistant Professor, Department of Otolaryngology – Head and Neck Surgery, Drexel University College of Medicine, Philadelphia, PA.

Bridget Rose, MM, MS, CCC-SLP, Instructor, Department of Otolaryngology – Head and Neck Surgery, Drexel University, College of Medicine, Philadelphia, PA.

Adam Rubin, M.D., Adjunct Assistant Professor, Michigan State University School of Medicine, Dept. of Otolaryngology – Head and Neck Surgery, University of Michigan Medical Center and Director, Lakeshore Professional Voice Center, Lakeshore Ear, Nose & Throat Center, St. Clair Shores, MI

John Rubin, M.D., F.A.C.S., F.R.C.S., Consultant Otolaryngologist, Royal National Throat, Nose and Ear Hospital; Honorary Senior Lecturer, University College London, London.

Robert T. Sataloff, M.D., D.M.A., F.A.C.S., Professor and Chairman, Department of Otolaryngology – Head and Neck Surgery and Senior Associate Dean for Clinical Academic Specialties, Drexel University College of Medicine, Philadelphia, PA.

Jeanna M. Stiadle, Ph.D., Department of Communication Sciences and Disorders, University of Wisconsin-Madison, Madison, WI.

Susan L. Thibeault, Ph.D., Department of Communication Sciences and Disorders, University of Wisconsin-Madison, Madison, and Division of Otolaryngology – Head & Neck Surgery, Department of Surgery, University of Wisconsin-Madison, Madison, WI.

Introduction

Jaime Eaglin Moore and Robert T. Sataloff.

The vocal fold is a complex layered structure as described by Minoru Hirano[1]. When vocal fold (VF) scar formation occurs, it disrupts the normal architecture of the lamina propria, and the mucosal wave is distorted affecting the quality of phonation. Alterations in the extracellular matrix, and particularly changes in the distribution of collagen, occur with scar formation. These changes affect the viscoelasticity of the vocal fold impairing the mucosal wave.

Many etiologies may cause scar including trauma (iatrogenic and non-iatrogenic), radiation, and inflammatory responses. Of particular concern to the otolaryngologist are iatrogenic causes. Gone are the days when vocal fold stripping was employed commonly. With advancements in phonosurgical techniques and increased understanding of the physiology of the vocal fold, post-operative voice outcomes have improved in the hands of experienced surgeons; but poor results do occur even in the best of hands.

Regardless of advancements in laryngeal microsurgery, vocal fold scar is still common in hoarse patients who present to the otolaryngologist's office. It is often missed on standard laryngoscopy, and the patient is frequently told his or her VFs are "normal on examination". Proper equipment such as strobovideolaryngoscopy and a trained practitioner are important in establishing the diagnosis of VF scar. Accurate diagnosis is crucial to devise an appropriate treatment plan that may include voice therapy and/or surgery. Accurate diagnosis also is needed to establish realistic expectations for the patient and surgeon.

Many treatment options are available for vocal fold scar from voice therapy to vocal fold reconstruction. Despite the advances in surgical technique and tissue engineering, vocal fold scar is a difficult disorder to treat, and outcomes of all treatments vary widely. The appropriateness of each management option for a patient depends upon the severity of the scar, dysphonia, and vocal effort, as well as the patient's needs. Knowledge of all treatment options and an understanding of the direction of future research are important for the clinician when approaching and counseling these challenging patients. We hope that the material summarized in this book will provide a broad perspective of the state-of-the-art in the diagnosis and treatment of scar that will be of practical value for the clinician.

Reference

1.   Hirano M, Kakita Y. Cover-body theory of vocal fold vibration. In: Daniloff R. (Ed.) *Speech Science: Recent Advances*. San Diego, CA: College-Hill Press; 1985.

Section I

Vocal fold anatomy and pathophysiology of scar

Jeanna M. Stiadle and Susan L. Thibeault

Introduction

According to estimates, at any given moment 20.7 million Americans have voice difficulties[1], and one of the primary reasons for dysphonia is vocal fold scar[2]. Vocal fold scar can cause vocal fatigue, hoarseness, and difficulty controlling the voice[3]. Treatment for vocal fold scar is limited secondary to a poor understanding of the biological mechanisms involved in this disorder. Scientists have begun investigating the cellular and molecular mechanisms involved in vocal fold scarring to better understand the complex processes involved in its manifestation[4]. More importantly, understanding these processes is necessary for clinicians as they strive to deliver effective treatments to ensure positive outcomes for their patients.

The introduction of scar to the lamina propria of the vocal fold has several complicated, lasting effects on its structure and function. Several main causes of scarring in the vocal fold have been identified. According to Benninger and colleagues[2], vocal fold scarring may be secondary to traumatic, neoplastic, iatrogenic, inflammatory, and miscellaneous etiologies.

Traumatic injuries are characterized by either blunt trauma or a type of penetrating injury. Neoplastic etiologies most commonly refer to scarring as a result of carcinoma on the vocal fold. Scarring due to a medical procedure such as an injection, prolonged intubation, or tracheotomy surgery is classified as iatrogenic. Inflammatory etiologies refer to scarring resulting from inflammatory conditions including gastroesophageal reflux disease and necrotizing infections. Other causes of vocal fold scar that do not correspond to the previous categories are noted as miscellaneous etiologies. The etiology can affect the scar's appearance and severity level[2].

Stages of wound healing

To be able to understand wound healing in the vocal folds, a review of the stages is presented. It should be noted that the majority of what is known regarding the stages of wound healing has been extrapolated from the skin literature. When injury occurs, tissue immediately begins the process of wound healing. The recognized stages of wound healing include coagulation, inflammation, mesenchymal cell (MSC) proliferation, angiogenesis, epithelization, protein synthesis, and contraction and remodeling. All of these stages contribute to changes in the epithelium and lamina propria leading to the eventual development of scar tissue. Although these stages are described separately, all are dependent on one another and can overlap[5].

During the first stage, coagulation, the body responds to extensive bleeding by forming a blood clot (hemostasis) at the site of the injury. After the clot is formed, the tissue undergoes alternating periods of vasoconstriction and vasodilation indicating the beginning of the inflammation stage. In the inflammation stage, neutrophils, albumin, and globulin infiltrate the matrix at the site of injury. Neutrophils are especially necessary to monitor and absorb foreign materials. Macrophages also emerge in the matrix and aid in tissue breakdown by secreting enzymes. MSC proliferation occurs days after coagulation and inflammation. This stage is characterized by the presence of fibroblasts at the site of the developing wound. Fibroblasts migrate across the wound site by binding and releasing substances such as fibronectin. Some fibroblasts undergo a change in phenotype to myofibroblasts to aid in the process of tissue repair. New blood vessels form at the site of the wound when several capillaries bind together signaling angiogenesis. The process of epithelialization results in a newly reformed epithelial barrier. At the edge of the wound, basal cells become thicker and migrate toward the collagen fibers present at the wound. Afterward, basal cells are restored to their previous phenotype.

The 'new' epithelium typically appears abnormal at the level of the dermis and epidermis as compared to an uninjured model. During protein synthesis, fibroblasts produce collagen at the wound site. Collagen forms a matrix to replace the previous fibrin scaffold allowing for cell movement. The last stage, contraction and remodeling, is the one in which scar tissue develops. This advanced stage can occur up to 12 months after the original injury.

Tissue is characterized by an increase in collagen density along the stress lines of the injury and the presence of metalloproteinases and enzymes at the site. As the remodeling stage progresses, collagen becomes less dense, and deposits of collagen bundles appear disorganized throughout the lamina propria. Elastin density also decreases, and fibers present as more short and compact than previously noted. Elastin, which promotes strength and flexibility, has an infrequent distribution in mature scars, never returning to baseline amounts[2].

Wound healing in the vocal fold epithelium

The layers that constitute the vocal mucosa are the epithelium, lamina propria, and deep muscle. Vocal fold epithelium is comprised of stratified squamous cells on the edge of the adducting folds[6]. The epithelium can be further subdivided into the suprabasal and basal layers. The epithelium contains a series of junctions that serve to connect epithelial cells to each other or to the matrix of the epithelium. There are three main types of cell junctions making up the epithelium: occluding (i.e. tight), anchoring, and communicating. Tight cell junctions are located near the edges of epithelial cells to seal the space between adjacent cells. These junctions mediate the cell's permeability. Anchoring junctions function similarly, in that they maintain strong bonds between cytoskeletons of adjacent cells or between cells and the basement membrane. Both tight and anchoring cell junctions serve to provide the epithelium with a barrier for protection of the vocal folds. Finally, communicating junctions allow electrical signaling between adjacent cells through ion transport. All three of these junctions are necessary to a functional epithelial layer[6].

In healthy human vocal folds, the epithelial cell layer is subjected to insult during everyday voice use. Savelli *et al.*[7] determined that the epithelium undergoes turnover once every 30 hours in a rat model under normal conditions. In order to maintain homeostasis and continue to provide protection to the vocal folds beneath it, the epithelium must be restored as quickly as possible. Leydon and colleagues[8] sought to determine the mechanism by which the epithelium maintains homeostasis and regenerates by identifying the density and location of stem cells within the epithelium. They found stem cells primarily in the stratified squamous epithelium along the length of the fold, suggesting that their principal function is to restore the cell layer along the part of the vocal fold most susceptible to damage[8].

The anatomy of the epithelium dictates its response during each stage of wound healing. Branski and colleagues[5] investigated the changes in the epithelial tissue during stages of early wound healing in a rabbit model. Immediately after the injury, the epithelium was absent; however, by the third day post-injury, proliferating inflammatory cells and fibroblasts at the site of the wound were observed, indicating the beginning of the inflammation stage. Next, new epithelial cells began proliferating at the site of the injury along with dense deposits of collagen. These observations are presumed to be part of the MSC proliferation and angiogenesis stages and were followed by dead epithelial cells being replaced by a new layer, signaling the epithelialization period.

Other studies have also targeted changes in the epithelium post-injury. Puchelle et al.[9] defined three main stages of epithelial regeneration following injury in airway epithelia: cell adhesion and migration, proliferation and stratification, and differentiation. Leydon et al.[10] later confirmed using a rat model that vocal fold epithelia follow this same pattern during post-injury regeneration. According to the study, cell adhesion and migration was evident 3 days post-injury. Epithelial proliferation was first observed one day after injury and continued through 5 days post-injury. Finally, a regenerated epithelium with differentiated cells was noted by day 15 post-injury. During the early stages of wound healing, Leydon and colleagues[10] noted the presence of EGF and TGFβ1 in the epithelial cells, suggesting that epithelial cells secrete these growth factors to mediate the process of regeneration. Leydon et al.[10] observed a restored epithelial barrier with intact intercellular junctions 3 days post-injury. However, a complete basement membrane was not observed until 5 weeks post injury. Despite the rapid structural restoration of the epithelial barrier, adequate functional restoration required additional time. Leydon and colleagues[10] observed leakiness in the epithelia until 2–5 weeks post-injury. The functional properties of the epithelial barrier are necessary for preventing the invasion of viruses, particulates, and bacteria into the vocal folds. Therefore, although structural aspects of the epithelial barrier may recover relatively soon after injury, more time may be important for functional properties to be restored.

Table 1.1 Stages of wound healing of the vocal fold—epithelium

Time point	Tissue changes	Corresponding stage
Immediately after	Epithelium appeared absent from sample[5]	N/A
3–5 days post-injury	Emerging epithelium Confluent, multilayered epithelium[10]	Cell adhesion and migration
1–15 days post-injury	Epithelial cell proliferation began 1 day after injury but was noted as sparse Proliferation peaked at 3 days and continued through day 5 New epithelial cells and collagen deposits at site Proliferation was complete by day 15	Proliferation and stratification MSC proliferation
5–15 days post-injury	Differentiated cells observed throughout epithelium Appears similar to uninjured control Full permeability of lamina propria still developing[10]	Differentiation

Wound healing in the lamina propria

The basement membrane of the epithelium separates it from the lamina propria (also known as Reinke's space), arguably the most complex section of the vocal folds. The uninjured lamina propria consists of fibrous proteins, such as collagen and elastin, and interstitial proteins. The extracellular matrix (ECM) forms the structure of the lamina propria. Each of the layers of the lamina propria have been characterized by unique concentrations of elastin and collagen. These layers include the superficial, intermediate, and deep layers. The superficial space is characterized by a predominance of reticular, elastic, and collagen fibers with relatively infrequent vocal fold fibroblasts. Macrophages and myofibroblasts are also present in this level of the lamina propria. The intermediate layer contains hyaluronic acid (HA) and fibromodulin. The number of elastic and collagen fibers increases moving toward the intermediate and deep layers of the lamina propria. The deep layer contains slightly less elastin than the intermediate layer and a similar concentration of collagen fibers. This layer also contains fibromodulin and HA.

The structure and function of interstitial proteins in the vocal folds are less well understood than the roles of collagen and elastin. However, these interstitial proteins may have a prominent role in oscillating the vocal folds. A proteoglycan has the ability to link to various types of molecules important to the function of vocal folds, such as water molecules. These proteins can control the concentration of carbohydrates and lipid molecules in the ECM thus affecting its biological properties. In addition, according to Gray, Titze, Chan, and Hammond[11], these proteins can support or suppress growth and modulate wound healing within the ECM. Large chain proteoglycans, such as HA, are important to viscosity, while small proteoglycans regulate collagen organization.

HA is an interstitial protein involved in the regulation of viscosity, flow, and dampening in the vocal folds[12]. In addition, it is recognized as contributing to wound healing without scar in models of fetal ECM[13]. However, not all studies have supported this proposed role of HA in wound healing. Thibeault *et al.*[3] investigated levels of collagen, elastin, and HA in normal and scarred vocal folds in a rabbit model. The investigation revealed less collagen and elastin in the scarred model, as expected. HA levels were not significantly different between the two models, suggesting that HA may not be as essential in wound healing of the vocal folds as originally hypothesized. On the other hand, HA derivative injectables have been shown to improve viscoelastic properties of the ECM when injected after surgery[14]. The exact function and contributions of HA in wound healing have yet to be fully understood.

Small proteoglycans include decorin, biglycan, and fibromodulin. Decorin is distributed in the superficial layer of the lamina propria, while fibromodulin is distributed in the middle and deep layers. Gray *et al.*[11] proposed that decorin may play a major role regulating fibroblasts as a response to injury. This theory would explain why superficial layers tend to show less overall damage after injury/surgery than the middle and deep layers where less decorin is present. In contrast, fibromodulin is responsible for the structure and function of tendons and ligaments during the wound-healing process. Glycoproteins are also involved in the regulation of the ECM during the wound-healing process. Fibronectin binds proteins and supplies strength to other cells in the ECM. This glycoprotein is present in normal vocal folds, but exists in elevated concentrations in scarred tissue.

Other cells in the ECM essential to wound healing include myofibroblasts and macrophages, both of which have been associated with synthesizing proteoglycans. Catten and collegues[16] found that in human vocal folds, myofibroblasts and macrophages appeared most frequently in the superficial portion of the lamina propria suggesting that these cells are involved with maintenance and repair before and after injury. Macrophages are specifically involved in conducting an inflammatory response. The authors of this study postulated that myofibroblasts contribute differently in the process of wound healing. Myofibroblasts were more prevalent than macrophages in the injured model and are linked to the processes of reorganization and repair in the vocal fold. The area of highest stress in the vocal folds (and likely the section most affected during injury) is the superficial layer of the lamina propria, which also has the highest concentration of myofibroblasts and macrophages.

Branski et al.[5] examined changes in the lamina propria throughout the wound-healing process using a rabbit model. Immediately after injury, the lamina propria appeared to be absent from the sample. A fibrinous blood clot formed 1 to 3 days after on the bed of the exposed muscle tissue, signaling the beginning of the coagulation stage. Evidence of a newly developing lamina propria was also observed in this area. By 3 to 10 days after injury, vascular channels appeared to form inside the lamina propria, signaling angiogenesis.

Hu et al.[15] described the process of wound healing in a canine model and specifically examined changes in concentrations of proteins in the ECM of the lamina propria using fluorescence. On day 15, increased collagen was observed in the ECM and remained until 6 months after injury. Elastin was observed throughout the lamina propria, but amounts decreased after the 15 day marker. By 6 months after injury, this decreased amount of elastin was noted in an irregular distribution in the lamina propria as compared to the control specimen. HA was distributed in the superficial and middle layers of the lamina propria in normal tissue[9], but was found throughout the lamina propria in the injured tissue at day 15. Similarly to elastin, amounts of HA decreased with time and by the 6-month marker less HA was noted in the injured tissue than in normal tissue.

Decorin was noted in the superficial layer of the lamina propria in the normal tissue, but was distributed throughout all layers of the lamina propria in the injured tissue. The concentration of decorin also decreased as the process of wound healing continued. By the 6-month time period, decorin in the injured tissue was significantly decreased as compared to the control[15].

Finally, fibronectin levels were found to be slightly increased in the injured tissue as compared to the control group. These changes in protein levels correspond to the different stages of wound healing. The increase in all of these proteins by day

15 suggests proliferation in the tissue related to the early wound-repair process. The increase in collagen noted at day 40 may correspond to the remodeling stage of the wound-healing process. Similar changes in these protein levels were described in a review by Hansen and Thibeault[17] who reviewed literature on rabbit, canine, rat, and pig models.

Table 1.2 Stages of wound healing of the vocal fold—lamina propria

Time point	Tissue changes	Corresponding stage
Immediately after–3 days post-injury	Lamina propria absent from sample[5] blood clot formed on surface of deep muscle over wound site[5]	N/A Coagulation
3–10 days post-injury	Inflammatory and fibroblast cells at site of injury[5] Vascular channels form within lamina propria[5]	Inflammation Angiogenesis
10–14 days post-injury	Disorganized pattern of collagen deposits and continued fibrosis[5]	Protein synthesis
15 days–6 months post-injury	Increased collagen observed in ECM Decreasing elastin throughout the lamina propria Increased HA[18,19] Increased decorin[19]	Contraction and remodeling
6 months–1 year post-injury	Decreased elastin[15]	

Other studies have shown contradictory results to Hu *et al.*[15] with regard to changes in HA and decorin during the wound-healing process. For example, a study investigating the role of HA in a rat model indicated that HA in scarred tissue remains at a higher level than normal tissue up to at least 2 months after injury[18]. In addition, Yamashita, Bless, and Welham[19] investigated gene concentrations in scarred and unscarred mouse vocal folds. They showed contradictory results in that HA and decorin both increased concentrations over time in scarred folds as compared to the controls. Therefore, despite Hu *et al.*[15] findings, more support exists for increases in HA and decorin rather than decreases[10].

Anatomy of a vocal fold scar

As previously stated, the final stage of the wound-healing process is scar formation. Scar tissue presents in a variety of anatomical forms with time: 1 to 3 months after the initial injury, early scar tissue develops. This type of scar is characterized by a stiff and thick quality. In contrast, a mature scar, one beyond 3 months old, is more thin and pliable than early scar. Injury to areas of tissue with higher levels of collagen and fibroblasts are more likely to lead to severe scarring[2].

In scar tissue, collagen, procollagen, and decorin increase in the ECM in an attempt to preserve the organization of collagen fibers. Fibronectin aids in adhesion and migration of these cells during repair. Finally, the increase of HA and loss of elastin contributes to increased stiffness and decreased viscosity in the lamina propria. Throughout the vocal fold, scar consists of disorganized collagen and elastin bundles, loss of constituents of the ECM, lower overall volume, and reduced pliability. The disorganized fibers contribute to distinct change in the biomechanical properties of voice[20]. The body–cover relationship is altered due to the consequences of the tissue injury, and the mucosal wave, which is essential to voice function, is severely compromised. The stiffer, less functional quality of the mucosal wave occurs as a result of the compromised concentration of elastin and collagen and the increased level of fibronectin.

Levels of viscoelasticity in vocal fold scar are especially important to treatment outcomes because the vocal folds are dependent on their ability to vibrate. Much research has examined properties of viscoelasticity in the vocal folds using a variety of models. Hertegerd and colleagues[21] examined properties of viscoelasticity in a rabbit model. They found that untreated vocal fold scar presented with longitudinally arranged fibrous bundles appearing similar to collagen. These bundles were not present in the uninjured vocal fold tissue. In addition, denser collagen was noted in the injured tissue than in the uninjured specimen. These numerous bundles and increased density of collagen likely contributed to an overall stiffer characterization in the scarred vocal fold.

Thibeault and colleagues[3] examined the changes in the lamina propria following the development of scar. Using a rabbit model, rheologic properties were examined to determine the modulus of elasticity and viscosity in the damaged tissue 2 months post-injury. Both stiffness and viscosity were significantly increased in the scarred model as compared to the uninjured model of the lamina propria. The decreased elasticity was presumably related to the scattered

NORMAL

SCARRED
(6 months - 1 year post-injury)

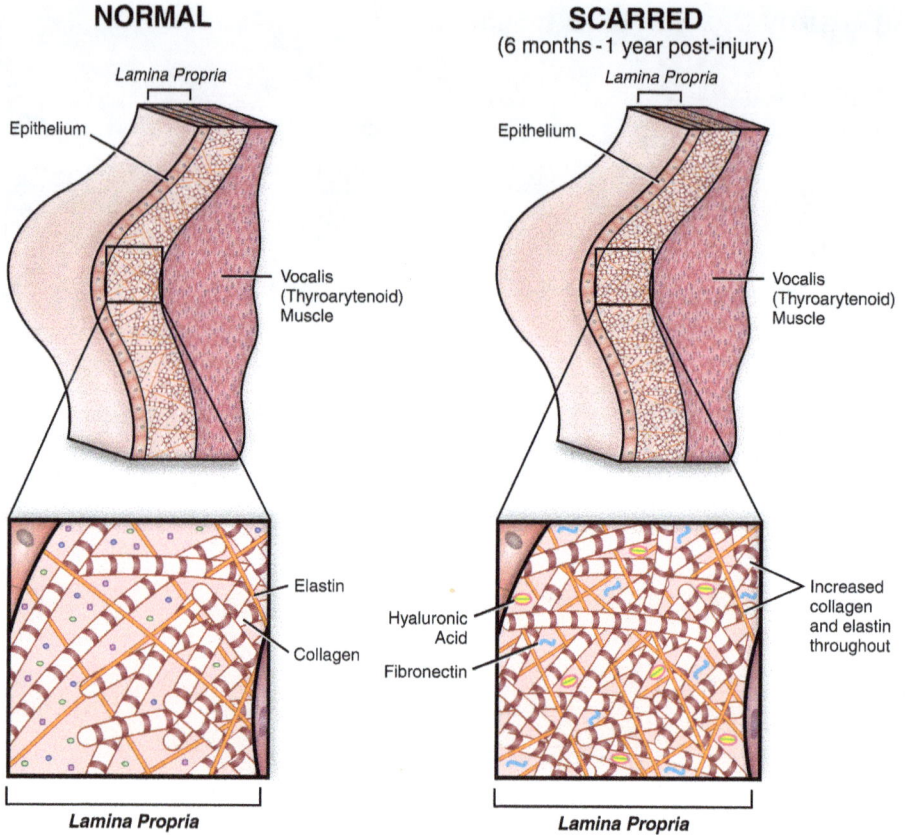

Figure 1.1 Schematic of normal and scarred vocal fold lamina propria. The scarred lamina propria is marked by an increase in collagen. The tissue is denser and thicker, causing decreased viscoelasticity and subsequent alteration of the mucosal wave propagation.

elastin fibers present in the scarred lamina propria. The difference in viscosity was also hypothesized as related to the change in the architecture of the fibers in the vocal folds. Hirschi and colleagues[22] also described fibronectin as a protein in the vocal folds that also may be related to increased viscosity in vocal fold scar.

Rousseau *et al.*[23] conducted a follow-up study to examine chronic scarring of the vocal folds in a rabbit model 6 months post-injury. Similarly, they found increased viscosity and increased modulus of elasticity in the scarred tissue as compared to normal tissue. Although other aspects of the tissue had returned to pre-injury levels (such as in collagen and procollagen), the disorganized elastin throughout the layers of the lamina propria persisted, likely contributing to the increased viscoelasticity in the scarred model. Rousseau *et al.*[23] also hypothesized that the observed higher density of the fibrous collagen bundles also contributed to increased viscoelasticity.

Cellular and molecular investigations: implications for prevention and treatment

Following injury, the vocal folds sustain many changes at the molecular level. Many studies have investigated means for prevention and treatment of these changes through cellular and molecular methodologies. These are discussed in more detail in a later chapter. Hirano et al.[24], for example, examined the use of growth factor therapy in treating vocal scarring in a canine model. They used hepatocyte growth factor (HGF), a polypeptide known to be involved in tissue regeneration of the liver and kidneys, and noted its effects on vocal fold vibrations in the scarred tissue of the canines via injection. Hirano et al.[25] had previously determined that use of HGF in vocal folds suppressed collagen production and increased the production of HA, suggesting a possible role in vocal fold wound healing. They found that the scarred vocal fold canine samples treated with HGF had overall better vibration according to the mucosal wave amplitude, suggesting that this treatment could reduce the negative effects of scarring on vocal fold vibration.

Some studies have used molecular work to prevent vocal fold scarring. Hirano et al.[25] used the previously described HGF injections in an acute rabbit model and measured its effects on vocal fold vibration and histological characteristics. In this study, they found that samples treated with HGF at the time of injury maintained a well-organized layer structure in the vocal fold with reduced collagen deposition as compared to the control group. In addition, the HGF treated samples did not exhibit tissue contraction of the lamina propria whereas the control did. Finally, results from the study indicated that HGF-treated samples were markedly less stiff, had less viscosity, and had better vibratory function than those in the control group. Results from this molecular study supported HGF therapy as a valid preventative technique in vocal fold wound healing.

A study by Chhetri et al.[26] used lamina propria replacement therapy with autologous fibroblasts as a technique for vocal fold scar treatment. They used a laser to create scar tissue on the vocal folds of canines and harvested tissue from the buccal cavities of the animals for tissue culture. Next, fourth passage cultured fibroblasts were injected into the scarred vocal folds of the canines.

Analysis revealed significant improvements in the mucosal waves and acoustic parameters following replacement therapy, showing promise for this method in future research.

Other studies have investigated the implementation of biomaterials in vocal fold rehabilitation. Jia *et al.*[27] developed HA-based soft microgels and cross-linked microgel networks for use in scarred vocal fold tissue in a canine model. The study determined that HA-based microgel networks can be constructed to have similar viscoelasticity to canine vocal fold tissue, indicating that these biomaterials would be useful in aiding in tissue regeneration.

Similarly, Hahn *et al.*[28] developed collagen-based microgel networks to examine their use in lamina propria regeneration. Scaffolds were comprised of collagen and HA or collagen and alginate, and pig vocal fold fibroblasts were added to the separate mixtures. The collagen–alginate hydrogels did not demonstrate scaffold compaction or loss of mass as compared to the collegen–HA hydrogels. In addition, the collagen–alginate hydrogels demonstrated ECM synthesis unlike the collagen–HA hydrogels in the study.

Xu *et al.*[29] developed a three-dimensional, biodegradable xenogeneic scaffold for the regeneration of vocal fold fibroblasts in the lamina propria using a decellularized bovine lamina propria. Results indicated that human vocal fold fibroblasts easily attached to the engineered acellular scaffold. High levels of decorin were noted as well as normal levels of viscoelasticity, which would potentially support vocal fold vibration in tissue generated from the scaffold.

Duflo *et al.*[30] engineered an HA–gelatin hydrogel to determine the appropriate amount of synthetic ECM necessary for wound repair in a rabbit model. HA hydrogels used in the study consisted of various gelatin concentrations. Analysis of gene expression revealed that all HA derived hydrogels, including the hydrogel without gelatin, resulted in increased tissue elasticity and viscosity. However, the HA hydrogel consisting of 5% gelatin showed the most improvement in all measured biomechanics in the study when injected immediately after injury.

More recent studies have examined the impact of architecture and other characteristics of proposed scaffolds on tissue regeneration and gene expression. Hughes and colleagues[31], for example, investigated the effects of aligned and unaligned electrospun scaffolds on vocal fold fibroblast behavior. Because vocal fold tissue is highly disorganized after scarring, it is important that treatment methods aim to reorganize this tissue during regeneration. Alignment of the ECM scaffold may play a role in the tissue's ability to reorganize. In this study, electrospinning was used to produce aligned and unaligned nanofibers for each of the scaffolds, and human vocal fold fibroblasts were seeded onto the scaffolds. Both aligned and unaligned scaffolds maintained a population of cells, but human vocal fibroblasts only oriented along the aligned scaffold. In addition, cell layers were arranged and confluent on the aligned scaffolds, but disorganized on the unaligned scaffolds.

Vocal fold scar results in numerous changes to the delicate anatomy of the vocal mechanism. These effects include physiological differences as well as changes in gene expression at molecular level of the lamina propria. Prevention and treatment must target where these changes occur in order to impact the structure and function of the vocal folds. Future research is necessary to determine viable treatment approaches for vocal fold scarring at the molecular level.

References

1. Roy N, Merrill RM, Gray SD, Smith EM. Voice disorders in the general population: prevalence, risk factors, and occupational impact. *Laryngoscope* 2005; 115:1988–1995.
2. Benninger MS, Alessi D, Archer S, *et al.* Vocal fold scarring: current concepts and management. *Otolaryngol Head Neck Surg.* 1996; 115(5):474–482.
3. Thibeault SL, Gray SD, Bless DM, *et al.* Histologic and rheologic characterization of vocal fold scarring. *J Voice* 2002; 16(1):96–104.
4. Benninger MS. Quality of the voice literature: What is there and what is missing? *J Voice* 2011; 25:647–652
5. Branski RC, Rosen CA, Verdolini K, Hebda PA. Acute vocal fold wound healing in a rabbit model. *Ann Otol Rhinol Laryngol* 2005; 114(1 Pt 1):19–24.
6. Levendoski EE, Leydon C, Thibeault SL. Vocal fold epithelial barrier in health and injury: A research review. *J Speech Lang Hear Res* 2014; 57(5):1679–1691.
7. Savelli V, Rizzoli R, Rizzi E, *et al.* Cell kinetics of vocal fold epithelium in rats. *Bollettino della Società italiana di biologia sperimentale* 1991; 67(12):1081–1088.
8. Leydon C, Bartlett R, Roenneburg D, Thibeault S. Localization of label-retaining cells in murine vocal fold epithelium. *J Speech Lang Hear Res* 2011; 54:1060–1066.
9. Puchelle E, Zahm JM, Tournier JM, Coraux C. Airway epithelial repair, regeneration, and remodeling after injury in chronic obstructive pulmonary disease. *Proc Am Thor Soc* 2006; 3:726–733.
10. Leydon C, Imaizumi M, Bartlett RS, *et al.* Epithelial cells are active participants in vocal fold wound healing: an in vivo animal model of injury. *PLoS ONE* 2014; 9(12):e115389. doi: 10.1371/journal.pone.0115389.
11. Gray SD, Titze IR, Chan R, Hammond TH. Vocal fold proteoglycans and their influence on biomechanics. *Laryngoscope* 1999; 109(6):845–854.

12. Ward PD, Thibeault SL, Gray SD. Hyaluronic acid: its role in voice. *J Voice* 2002; 16(3):303–309.
13. Moriarty KP. Hyaluronic acid-dependent pericellular matrices in fetal fibroblasts: Implications for scar-free wound repair. *Wound Repair Regen* 1996; 4:346–352
14. Hansen JK, Thibeault SL, Walsh JF, *et al.* In vivo engineering of the vocal fold extracellular matrix with injectable hyaluronic acid hydrogels: early effects on tissue repair and biomechanics in a rabbit model. *Ann Otol Rhinol Laryngol* 2005; 114:662–670.
15. Hu R, Xu W, Ling W, *et al.* Characterization of extracellular matrix proteins during wound healing in the lamina propria of vocal fold in a canine model: a long-term and consecutive study. *Acta Histochem* 2014; 116(5):730–735.
16. Catten M, Gray SD, Hammond TH, *et al.* Analysis of cellular location and concentration in vocal fold lamina propria. *Otolaryngol Head Neck Surg* 1998; 118(5):663–667.
17. Hansen JK, Thibeault SL. Current understanding and review of the literature: vocal fold scarring. *J Voice* 2006; 20(1):110–120.
18. Tateya I, Tateya T, Watanuki M, Bless DM. Homeostasis of hyaluronic acid in normal and scarred vocal folds. *J Voice* 2014; 29(2):133–139.
19. Yamashita M, Bless DM, Welham NV. Morphological and extracellular matrix changes following vocal fold injury in mice. *Cells Tissues Organs* 2010; 192:262–271.
20. Sataloff RT. *Professional Voice: The Science and Art of Clinical Care* 3 edn. San Diego: Plural Publishing Inc. 2005.
21. Hertegård S, Cedervall J, Svensson B, *et al.* Viscoelastic and histologic properties in scarred rabbit vocal folds after mesenchymal stem cell injection. *Laryngoscope* 2006; 116(7):1248–1254.
22. Hirschi SD, Gray SD, Thibeault SL. Fibronectin: an interesting vocal fold protein. *J Voice* 2002; 16(3):310–316.
23. Rousseau B, Hirano S, Scheidt TD, *et al.* Characterization of vocal fold scarring in a canine model. *Laryngoscope* 2003; 113(4):620–627.
24. Hirano S, Bless D, Heisey D, Ford C. Roles of hepatocyte growth factor and transforming growth factor beta1 in production of extracellular matrix by canine vocal fold fibroblasts. *Laryngoscope* 2003; 113:144–148.
25. Hirano SH, Bless DM, Nagai H, *et al.* Growth factor therapy for vocal fold scarring in a canine model. *Ann Otol Rhinol Laryngol* 2004; 113:777–785.
26. Chhetri DK, Head C, Revazova E, *et al.* Lamina propria replacement therapy with cultured autologous fibroblasts for vocal fold scars. *Otolaryngol Head Neck Surg* 2004; 131(6):864–870.
27. Jia X, Yeo Y, Clifton RJ, *et al.* Hyaluronic acid-based microgels and microgel networks for vocal fold regeneration. *Biomacromolecules* 2006; 7(12):3336–3344.
28. Hahn MS, Teply BA, Stevens MM, *et al.* Collagen composite hydrogels for vocal fold lamina propria restoration. *Biomaterials* 2006; 27(7):11041109.
29. Xu C, Chan RW, Tirunagari N. A biodegradable, acellular xenogeneic scaffold for regeneration of the vocal fold lamina propria. *Tissue Eng* 2007; 13(3):551566.

30. Duflo S, Thibeault SL, Li W, *et al*. Vocal fold tissue repair in vivo using a synthetic extracellular matrix. *Tissue Eng* 2006; 12(8):2171–2180.
31. Hughes LA, Gaston J, McAlindon K, *et al*. Electrospun fiber constructs for vocal fold tissue engineering: Effects of alignment and elastomeric polypeptide coating. *Acta Biomater* 2014; 13:111–120.

2

Diagnosis of vocal fold scar

Hayley Herbert and John Rubin

Introduction

The accurate diagnosis of vocal fold scar requires a multidisciplinary, systematic approach. Scarring of the vocal fold presents with a diverse range of symptoms and signs and should be considered in the differential diagnosis of any dysphonic patient. Diagnosing scar requires a high index of suspicion as the absence of normal vibratory tissue is often more difficult to detect than other pathology.

Vocal fold scar occurs when the lamina propria of the vocal fold becomes damaged. This is often associated with loss of critical extracellular matrix components, volume deficiency and reduced pliability[1] that interferes with the mobility and/or integrity of the layers of the vocal fold, impairing the mucosal wave and resulting in dysphonia. In accordance with source-filter theory described by Fant[2], alterations to vocal fold vibration affect the acoustic signal. The vast majority of these changes that affect the acoustic signal occur in the cover of the vocal fold. Scarring may also result in incomplete glottic closure thereby increasing vocal symptoms.

Causes of scarring

Acquired injury is the most common cause of vocal fold scarring. Congenital causes such as sulcus vocalis should also be considered, in particular in cases such as monocorditis, or long-standing hoarseness with secondary evidence of muscle tension.

Possible causes include those listed in Table 2.1.

Table 2.1 Causes of vocal fold scarring

Mechanism	Examples
Phonotrauma	Overuse, misuse
Chemical	Smoking, laryngopharyngeal reflux
Thermal	Laser, diathermy, inhalational
Trauma	Blunt and penetrating
Surgery	All vocal fold surgery, intubation, radiotherapy, injection laryngoplasty
Inflammatory	Systemic Lupus Erythematosus (SLE), Sjogrens, Rheumatoid Arthritis, scleroderma
Infective	Papilloma, bacterial laryngitis
Cancer	Squamous cell cancer, adenocarcinoma, adenoid cystic cancer
Vascular	Arteriovenous malformations, varices, telangiectasia
Congenital	Sulcus vocalis, congenital cyst

Phonotrauma

Phonotrauma typically impacts the basement membrane of the epithelium and the superficial layer of the lamina propria (SLLP). Dikkers *et al*[3] have studied benign lesions with electron microscopy and demonstrated deposition of electron-dense matter with loss of normal hemidesmosomes and anchoring fibers. They associated this with vibratory stress.

Gray and colleagues[4] have posited patterns of injury on the basis of immuno-histochemistry as follows:

1. Basement Membrane Zone (BMZ) and SLLP disruption with disorganization of the anchoring fibers and increased fibronectin, which they cited as being almost unique to the vocal fold and suggestive of a repetitive injury.

2. BMZ relatively intact, but a paucity of structural glycoproteins and interstitial proteins in the SLLP, as seen in certain cases of Reinke's edema and polyps.

Rubin and Yanagisawa[5] reported that the majority of phonotrauma occurs at the mid-membranous vocal fold, as this is the locus of greatest stress during normal phonation. Vocal overuse or more specifically misuse may result in vocal scarring in this region.

Chemical

Cigarette smoke and laryngopharyngeal reflux are irritants that can cause injury to the vocal folds (including the formation of Reinke's edema) whereby the normal structures of the epithelium and SLLP are altered. This may later form a vocal fold scar with fibrosis of the layers of the fold.

Thermal

Thermal injury to the vocal folds can be inflicted on surrounding normal tissues as the energy is transmitted into the subepithelial layers. Thermal damage also may occur beyond the edge of the cut, which is usually regarded as the margin of excision. The spot size, tissue relaxation time and energy delivered should all be carefully adjusted to achieve the desired function (e.g. incision or coagulation) with minimal damage to the normal tissues of the vocal fold. Diathermy similarly needs to be appropriately adjusted to reduce collateral damage and potential scar. The size and anatomic position of the larynx make it susceptible to inhalational injury. Smoke and steam burns can cause immediate and delayed damage to the larynx. Life-threatening edema can result from inhalational burns – especially steam, which has a heat capacity 4000 times that of air. Delayed scarring may result from this damage.

Trauma

Blunt and penetrating injuries to the larynx may lead to disruption to the laryngeal framework, webbing within the glottis, and injuries to the vocal folds as a result of the initial trauma, associated hemorrhage or infection.

Surgery

Post-operative dysphonia can be related to a number of factors including the:

- type and extent of the lesion,
- amount of fibrosis and scar involving the epithelium and Reinke's layers,
- amount of surgical dissection, and
- extent of epithelial resection and the resultant secondary healing processes[6].

Bouchayer and Cornut have identified four clinical patterns of post-operative vocal fold scar[7]. They have classified them into notches, webs, fibrous scars, and vocal fold rigidity.

Inflammatory

Vocal fold changes have been associated with systemic inflammatory disease such as systemic lupus erythematous (SLE). Bamboo nodes (primary vocal fold lesions associated with autoimmune disease) have been shown to contain extensive fibrinoid necrosis surrounded by a rim of histiocytes in a palisading fashion[8].

Infection

Human Papilloma Virus (especially HPV subtypes 6 and 11) can be clinically expressed as florid Recurrent Respiratory Papillomatosis. Management of these lesions may lead to significant scarring and webbing within the larynx. Surgical treatment for other types of airway or voice compromise also has a risk of vocal fold scarring. Laryngitis caused by granulomatous infections, such as tuberculosis and syphilis, may result in scarring.

Cancer

Most laryngeal cancer is caused by squamous cell carcinoma. Less common malignant tumors that affect the larynx include adenocarcinoma, adenoid cystic, or chondrosarcoma. Destruction and distortion of the normal tissues of the larynx by the cancer or by the oncological management treatments (including surgery, radiotherapy and/ or chemotherapy) may result in vocal fold scarring.

Vascular

Disruption of the normal tissue planes by vascular anomalies, resultant hemorrhages, and the treatment of these may result in scarring.

Congenital

Developmental absence of tissue – such as sulcus vocalis or congenital epidermoid cysts – may result in scarring of the vocal folds.

Sulcus vocalis

Sulcus vocalis can be both congenital and acquired. This is addressed in Chapter 7 but can present in a similar manner to post-traumatic scarring.

Ford[9] classified sulcus into three types:

1. *Physiologic sulcus*: superficial depression on the vocal fold not affecting mucosal wave.

2. *Sulcus vergeture*: atrophic changes in the vocal fold epithelium. This epithelium is not attached to the vocal ligament and symptoms are not as severe as they are in sulcus vocalis. Patients may be asymptomatic.

3. *Sulcus vocalis*: in this condition the superficial layer of the lamina propria is absent altogether or a portion of the epithelium invaginates through the superficial layer of the lamina propria and adheres to the vocal ligament.

There is an increase in collagen fibers and deficiency of capillaries in the region of the sulcus. Sulcus results in stiffness of the vibratory margin of the vocal folds, and often in adynamic segments. This produces dysphonia, with breathiness, increased phonation threshold pressure and voice fatigue.

Patient evaluation

The team

A voice team should include an otolaryngologist and speech language pathologist. In centers with a specialized voice laboratory, a voice scientist may be involved. Additional members of the team may include specialists from neurology, psychology, physiotherapy and pedagogy.

This integrated holistic assessment of the patient with vocal fold scarring will facilitate improved accuracy of diagnosis and contribute to the formulation of a treatment plan.

Self-evaluation questionnaires should be used routinely to facilitate individual-ized patient diagnosis and treatment plans. Logistically these can be completed in the waiting room or prior to arrival. This is also helpful to gain some idea of the current vocal handicap. There are several options to choose from including the Voice Handicap Index (VHI)[10]. The VHI-10 is a validated 10-question adaption of the original questionnaire[11].

History

Practitioners need to understand the present voice complaint and the impact this problem has on the patient's daily life. The age and gender of the patient should be established as well as the occupation and vocal requirements.

Patients with clinically significant vocal fold scarring may have a diverse range of symptoms. Typically these are a combination of dysphonia, vocal fatigue, loss of vocal control, and breathiness[12]. Patients' symptoms vary because scar tissue contains a large amount of disorganized collagen bundles. This impacts upon the pliability of the epithelium and the viscoelastic character of the SLLP. The mass, stiffness, and vocal closure will vary in relation to the degree, extent, and location of injury. The location of adynamic areas within the fold may vary thus influencing the overall acoustic output.

Specific questions required during history taking include:

- Duration of symptoms and onset.
- Problematic activities (e.g. warm up times, singing voice, talking, shouting).
- Factors that improve or worsen the symptoms.
- Current vocal demands.
- Current assessment of vocal disability.*

Discussion points with the patient should include:

- Previous intubations and duration.
- Surgeries both non-laryngeal and laryngeal. For laryngeal surgeries, operation notes and pictures are helpful.

---

* This will be assisted by their perception based VHI score.

23

- Any trauma to the head and neck.
- Exposure to chemicals or gases (occupational or social).
- Smoking history.
- History of reflux and severity.
- History of cancer.
- Previous radiation therapy.
- Excessive, forceful, or unusual speaking and singing styles.
- Background medical history, in particular looking for underlying inflammatory conditions and neurologic diseases.

A complete medical and medication (both prescription and over the counter) history should be documented at the first consultation.

Examination

Perceptual

When taking a patient's history it is important to grade the patient's current level of dysphonia. The most widely used and accepted scale for auditory–perceptual evaluation is the GRBAS scale[13] (Table 2.2).

Table 2.2 GRBAS scale for evaluating the hoarse voice

Parameter	Definition (Hirano)
Grade (G)	Overall severity
Roughness (R)	Psychoacoustic impression of irregular vocal-fold vibration
Breathiness (B)	Psychoacoustic impression of air leakage through the glottis
Asthenia (A)	Weakness or lack of power in voice
Strain (S)	Psychoacoustic impression of a hyperfunctional state of phonation

Each parameter is given a severity score of 0–3. The grade is the overall or worst score.

Source: From Hirano M. Psycho-acoustic evaluation of voice: GRBAS scale for evaluating the hoarse voice. *Clinical Examination of the Voice*. New York: Springer-Verlag; 1981.

Objective assessments

Voice laboratory measurements are the gold standard for quantitative assessment of voice – these will be discussed later. However, a basic acoustic assessment can be performed in the office using a number of devices such as Visi-Pitch (Visi-Pitch, KayPentax, Montvale, NJ, USA).

The senior author (JR) routinely uses the mobile Application "OperaVox." This information can be gathered on an iPhone or similar device in the office or on the ward pre-operatively. If a full acoustic analysis is not available this is a useful tool for diagnosis and for measurement of change with treatment. It includes measurements of fundamental frequency, shimmer (cycle-to-cycle variation in energy or amplitude), jitter (cycle-to-cycle variation in duration), range, and maximum phonatory time. It has recently been shown to be comparable to *Multi-Dimensional Voice Program*™ [14] (MDVP, KayPentax, Montvale, NJ, USA).

Physical examination

A directed examination of the head and neck should be performed in all patients:

- *Ear exam*: chronic hearing loss may result in inappropriate loudness of voice causing phonotrauma. An audiogram should be performed and ears examined.

- *Nose exam*: chronic nasal and sinus disease may result in irritation of the larynx. Allergy may also cause microtrauma to the larynx and thus signs of this should be assessed. Nasal examination is advised.

- *Oral cavity*: dental hygiene, xerostomia, and oral health should be assessed as possible contributing factors to the patient's dysphonia. Wear of dental enamel may be a sign of laryngopharyngeal reflux.

- *Neck*: inspection of the neck is useful to assess any scarring from trauma or surgery. The patient's neck should be examined for increased muscle tension and movement of the larynx on phonation. Excessive muscle tension is frequently seen as a byproduct of adaptation to vocal fold stiffness as well as other vocal fold pathology. Mathieson *et al*[15] have devised a protocol for assessment of muscle tension. The thyroid should also be palpated.

The mirror examination of the vocal folds has to some degree been superseded as a technique for viewing the larynx. This is unfortunate as it allows the most natural appreciation of the "true" color of the vocal folds and is still the baseline evaluation of a number of laryngologists[16].

The two main techniques for viewing the vocal folds in the office include rigid laryngoscopy and flexible nasolaryngoendoscopy. The use of rigid or flexible scopes with high-definition monitors allows good resolution images of the surface of the folds to be displayed.

Rigid laryngoscopy involves the use of a wide-bore rigid angled endoscope. The patient is seated comfortably. Feet should be planted on the floor. If able, the patient will flex the neck on the shoulders and extend the head, open the mouth and extend the tongue to be held by either the examiner or patient. The patient is instructed to give a slight smile imagining he or she is biting into an apple and at the same time phonate a medium and high frequency "heeee." The scope should be gently advanced to avoid any surface contact with the posterior oral cavity. Excellent views of the vocal folds can often be gained.

A study has shown that rigid endoscopy provides superior images of the true vocal folds, necessary for precise diagnosis in patients with true vocal fold pathology[17]. Thus, if tolerated, rigid endoscopy for the diagnosis of vocal fold scar is preferred. However this technique can be limited in patients with a large tongue, active gag reflex, and patients with severe trismus.

In these cases a distal chip-tip flexible endoscope may be used. The patient is seated as above. Local anesthetic can be used in the nose if required. The scope can be passed either between the middle and inferior turbinate or along the floor of the nasal cavity. This technique usually affords a longer examination of the vocal folds, and allows the patient to use the voice in continuous speech and even in song. This is particularly helpful if adynamic portions of the vocal fold are suspected, and is a boon to identifying vocal fold fibrosis.

If a diagnosis of vocal fold scarring is suspected, the best equipment suitable for patient and examiner should be used as it must be appreciated that some scarring is subtle and may be difficult to identify. The aim of examination should be to achieve clear detail of the surface of the vocal folds. The examination should also be recorded and played back in real time and slow motion to detect any abnormality with white light. Abnormal vasculature or change in color on the superficial surface of the folds may alert the examiner to the site of the scar. Abnormal supraglottic muscle tension and ventricular adduction may be a secondary phenomenon of the scar, and thus the vocal fold mucosal surfaces require close inspection and exclusion of pathology before a primary diagnosis of dysphonia related to muscle tension is made.

Stroboscopy is endoscopy performed with an intermittent light flashing at a predetermined frequency or a frequency synchronized to the patient's fundamental frequency of phonation. It involves judgments and ratings of a series of parameters such as glottic closure, symmetry, regularity, and mucosal wave. All of these parameters may be affected by vocal scar. They can be rated using a grading scale[18].

- *Glottal closure:* the medial edge of the affected vocal fold may not meet the contralateral fold or the fold may be at different levels and result in a glottic gap.

- *Mucosal wave:* there may be a localized decreased mucosal amplitude and mucosal wave present. A completely adynamic segment may be present on the side of vocal fold scar.

- *Vocal fold symmetry:* this entails a rating of the comparative motion of both folds. Asymmetry is likely to be caused by reduction in vibratory capacity of one fold – such as a vocal fold scar.

- *Regularity*: degree of irregular slow motion may be assessed.

Classification of scar severity

A common clinical feature of scarring is a spindle-shaped glottis during phonation with insufficient closure and air leakage and impaired vocal fold vibration with reduced amplitude and reduced or mostly absent mucosal wave. Vibrations are mostly asymmetric and irregular[12]. Scarring frequently causes areas of adynamism and interferes with the mucosal wave. Thus it may alter phonation by mechanical restriction or impact on closure. It must also be recalled that there may be scar affecting the cricoarytenoid joint, for example in cases of rheumatoid arthritis or trauma, and this may have a further impact upon the ability of the vocal folds to form a seal[20].

Arens and Remacle[19] have classified the severity of scar formation into four types:

- *Type I*: mild to moderate glottis insufficiency and reduced vibration of the vocal folds. The scar involves the mucosal and submucosal levels of the vocal fold.

- *Type II*: anterior moderate glottis insufficiency seen around the anterior commissure region with no vibrations of the vocal folds. The scar involves the vocalis muscle.

- *Type III*: considerable glottis insufficiency and rotated arytenoid may be noted. The scar formation is adherent to the inner perichondrium and the cartilage, and the defect extends up to the supraglottic region

- *Type IV*: considerable glottis insufficiency with bilaterally reduced vibration of the vocal folds. Web formation is found at the anterior commissure region.

Investigations

Voice laboratory

A voice laboratory is a requirement for all practitioners conducting research on voice. It can be useful clinically for objectively quantifying the vocal fold scar's impact and monitoring any changes following rehabilitation.

Acoustic analysis

Essential to the diagnosis of vocal scar and sulcus vocalis is reliable and valid voice assessment. Acoustic analysis is a non-invasive objective method of assessing voice quality. Recordings of speaking and singing voice are taken either in analog or digital form. If analog, these are converted to a digital format (analog to digital or A/D conversion) and acoustic parameters are measured and analyzed using sophisticated voice software.

Appropriate technical and procedural protocols should be followed to ensure the integrity and repeatability of data collected for acoustic analysis[21]. A professional grade microphone should be used at a distance of 3–4 cm, 45–90 degrees from the mouth. Ambient noise and room reverberation should be minimized (a soundproof room is ideal). Data should be directly digitized to computer or stored using digital audio tape technology.

Normative data have been established for acoustic measures, against which the results can be compared. These measures reflect the state of the larynx and do not necessarily diagnose a specific disorder.

Analyses can be used to determine fundamental frequency, harmonic spectrum, jitter (frequency perturbation), shimmer (amplitude perturbation), signal to noise ratio (SNR), harmonic to noise ratio (HNR), breathiness index and other parameters. These measures can be calculated using popular commercial voice assessment programs such as the *Multidimensional Voice Program* (MDVP, Kay Pentax, Montvale, NJ, USA) and *Dr Speech* (Tiger DRS Inc., Seattle, WA, USA).

A phonetogram of the frequency range at varying intensities of voice can be drawn. It is, however, very time consuming. Sound spectrography or the resolution of a periodic waveform into a series of sine waves of different frequencies, amplitudes, and phase relationships can be performed.

Most disorders of the larynx do not appear to have a significant influence on mean speaking fundamental frequency (F_0); however, F_0 variability and range do seem to reflect tissue changes[22].

The main limitation of traditional acoustic analysis algorithms stems from their dependency on near-periodic signals[23]. Titze[24] described a consensus workshop on acoustic analysis that suggests adoption of signal types to ensure that normal and disordered voices are appropriately analyzed. See Table 2.3. Vocal fold scarring and pathologic sulcus vocalis patients predominantly exhibit type 2 and 3 voice signals[25].

Table 2.3 Voice signal types and appropriate analysis

Type	Definition	Appropriate Analysis
Type 1	Near periodic signals	Time-domain based perturbation analyses
Type 2	At least one qualitative signal bifurcation	Visual displays such as spectrograms or reconstructed phase plots
Type 3	Complete aperiodicity/ chaos	Auditory-perceptual ratings or nonlinear dynamic parameters

Source: Voice signal types and appropriate analysis. From Titze IR. *Workshop on Acoustic Voice Analysis: Summer Statement.* Iowa City IA: National Center for Voice and Speech; 1995.

Nonlinear methods – such as correlation dimension, phase space reconstruction, or Lyapunov exponents – have shown promise in clinical voice analysis as they are able to analyze irregular and chaotic oscillations[26,27]. Jiang *et al*[28] emphasized that perturbation measures and nonlinear dynamic analysis provide complementary information. Using a combination of perturbation measures with nonlinear methods can provide more precise results, especially in analysis and description of patients with severe voice disorders.

Another method of analyzing the aperiodic voice signal in vocal fold scar is Cepstral Peak Prominence (CPP). CPP measure is the difference in amplitude between the cepstral peak and the corresponding value on the regression line that is directly below the peak (i.e. the predicted magnitude for the frequency at the cepstral peak). The CPP measure represents how far the cepstral peak emerges from the cepstrum background[29]. This is a measure of the degree of harmony within a voice sample. It has several advantages as a measure of dysphonia:

1. It does not rely on pitch tracking and therefore produces valid and reproducible values even for very aperiodic signals.
2. It is not dependent on recording technique or affected by differences in the volume of the voice sample being measured
3. It is presently the measure that correlates best with perceptual measures of dysphonia compared with other objective voice measures[30].

Aerodynamic measures

Aerodynamic measures provide an analysis of respiratory function, airflow pressures, and the characteristics of airflow from the patient.

Tidal volume, functional residual capacity, inspiratory capacity, total lung capacity, vital capacity, forced vital capacity, forced expiratory volume, and maximal mid-expiratory volume are basic pulmonary tests that can be measured in most voice laboratories.

Studies of airflow efficiency offer valuable information to physicians. Four parameters measured traditionally in the laboratory are

1. subglottal pressure,
2. supraglottal pressure,
3. glottal impedance, and
4. volume velocity of airflow at the glottis.

In the standard method, subglottal air pressure estimates are based on intra-oral air pressure measurements that are obtained during vocal fold abduction indicated by lip closure during production of the p-sound. This method works because air pressure equilibrates throughout the airway (subglottal pressure = intraoral air pressure).

Different calculations can determine:

1. mean flow rate (MFR),

2. glottal resistance, and

3. phonation quotient (PQ).

The mean value of the airflow rate at the glottis during sustained phonation is assessed for clinical purposes and is called the mean airflow rate (MFR).

PQ is defined as the vital capacity divided by the maximum phonation time (MPT). Because the total air volume consumed during maximum sustained phonation is less than the vital capacity, PQ is usually larger than MFR[31].

The minimum level of lung pressure needed to sustain vocal fold oscillation at a specific pitch is referred to as the phonation threshold pressure (PTP). Mathematical and physical laryngeal models have demonstrated that phonation threshold pressures are sensitive to vocal fold thinning, viscous shear properties of the tissue, and vocal tract inertance[32].

In a patient with vocal fold scarring the pulmonary function tests are often not specifically affected. Subglottic pressures, however, may not be maintained due to glottis gap.

Microlaryngoscopy

Microlaryngoscopy with palpation of the scarred larynx and/or palpation under high magnification has a role in assessment of vocal fold scar. This diagnostic procedure will not be required in all presenting patients. However, should voice analysis indicate pathology and there is no visual evidence of this, then microlaryngoscopy is recommended. The advantages of a diagnostic microlaryngoscopy include the following.

1. Superior microscopic views of all surfaces of the vocal folds. This includes infracordal views with a 70 or 90 degree angled Hopkins rod. Difficult diagnoses such as mucosal bridges and sulcus vocalis are easier to make using this technique.

2. Examination of the subglottis and trachea can be performed.

3. Vocal folds and cricoarytenoid joints can be palpated and manipulated.

4. It allows for "mapping out" of the lesion.

5. It allows for infiltration of normal saline under the epithelium of the vocal fold. See Figure 2.1. This gives information regarding the severity of scarring and amount of tethering of the epithelium to the vocal fold ligament. It will allow classification of sulcus vocalis and give an indication of likelihood of success of surgical intervention for the scar.

6. This examination also allows the surgeon to determine the type of access (i.e. which laryngoscope) the patient's anatomy will allow, information important for surgical treatment.

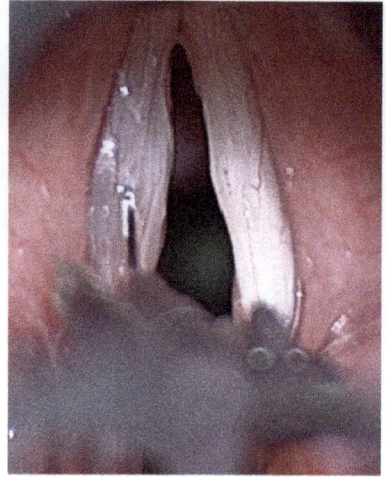

Figure 2.1: Infiltration of saline during microlaryngoscopy to investigate the extent of sulcus vocalis.

To a lesser or greater degree, this information can also be obtained with the patient awake and the larynx adequately anesthetized with local anesthetic agents.

Advanced vocal fold imaging

Stroboscopy allows an excellent estimation of vocal fold vibration when the vocal fold cycles are regular. However the flashes of light will not be synchronized with the vocal fold cycle if the vibrations are irregular and therefore more advanced systems are important to accurately examine the mucosal wave.

High-speed digital imaging

This modality allows accurate assessment of vocal fold movement. Although initially introduced in the late 1930s[33], the technology has not been adopted en masse as vast amounts of data are produced requiring sophisticated analysis. However, as digital image processing systems improve, becoming more powerful and easier to access, high-speed digital image technology has become more commonly utilized.

The process of capturing the images is similar to videolaryngoscopy, but it is more common for the rigid endoscope to be used. Traditional videolaryngoscopy is captured at a rate of 25–40 frames per second compared with 2000–8000 frames per second with high-speed laryngoscopy. In keeping with this the mucosal surface detail of the vocal fold is far superior to standard stroboscopy. The huge amount of data generated means that high-speed digital imaging is limited by the sampling rate to a few seconds. After acquisition of the images, transfer and computer analysis of the data can take several minutes. Review of a 2-second sample of the images can take close to 7 minutes[33]. See Figure 2.2.

Acoustic signals should be captured simultaneously to allow meaningful analysis of the relationship between vocal fold vibration and phonation.

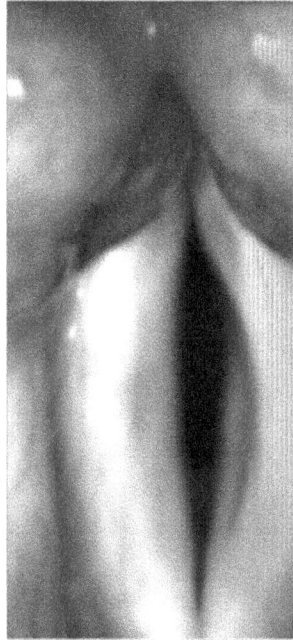

Figure 2.2: Still image of HSDI from a patient with right VF scar showing minimal vibratory amplitude and no mucosal wave on the scarred side compared to the non-scarred left side. Printed with permission from Dr Nathan Welham.

Videokymography

This method revived the principle of kymographic imaging, which displays the vibrations of the vocal folds and the surrounding tissues in a single image. The vocal folds are scanned and several successive glottal cycles are represented in the image. Schutte and Svec[34] developed videokymography to observe vocal fold movement. The system uses a modified video camera that works in two modes: a normal video camera, recording 50 images/second, and videokymographic mode, which can record images from a single, selected transverse line at approximately 8000 Hz. The successive line images are presented in real time on a monitor in such a way that the time dimension is displayed in a vertical direction, replacing the original spatial dimension. The resulting kymographic image, which shows the vibrations of the selected part of the vocal folds, enriches stroboscopy and enables the analysis of aperiodic vibration, particularly helpful in patients with vocal fold scarring. See Figure 2.3a and b.

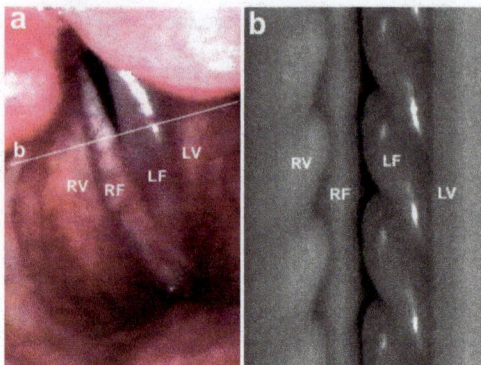

Figure 2.3: Strobolaryngoscopic (a) and videokymographic (b) images of a male larynx with scarred right vocal fold (RF) and chronic edema on the left vocal fold (LF). The videokymographic image was obtained from the position marked by the line in (a). In (b), notice the absence of vibrations on the scarred right vocal fold (RF) in contrast to the left vocal fold (LF), which vibrates. The right ventricular fold (RV) reveals vibrations of the same frequency and similar amplitude as the left vocal fold (LF). The left ventricular fold (LV) does not vibrate. Total time displayed in the videokymogram is 18.4 ms. (Image courtesy of Drs. J.G. Svec and F. Sram. For more details, see the publication Svec JG, Sram F, and Schutte HK. Videokymography. In: *The Larynx*. Third Edition. Volume I, edited by Fried MP and Ferlito A. San Diego, CA: Plural Publishing, 2009; and Svec JG, Sram F, and Schutte HK. Videokymography in voice disorders: What to look for? *Ann Otol Rhinol Laryngol* 116: 172–180, 2007).

Optical coherence tomography (OCT)

This is a noncontact noninvasive technology that measures light backscattered from within tissue to provide cross-sectional images of architecture. It has the ability to resolve subepithelial tissue microstructure[35]. It is based around a similar principle to ultrasound, using interferometric methods to detect light reflected up to 2 mm within tissue. By comparing the way light is polarized within the tissues to how it is reflected on the surface polarization-sensitive images are formed. Because these images detect orientation of collagen fiber bundles and can delineate lamina propria layers this technology shows promise to diagnose the disruption of the lamina propria present in vocal fold scarring[36].

Narrow band imaging/iScan

High-resolution digital chromoendoscopy can be performed using either pre- or post-processed systems. Pre-processed Narrow band imaging (NBI) (Olympus, Waltham, MA) and post-processed iScan (Pentax Medical Company, Montvale, NJ) are the two main systems used. This technology provides an additional filter that narrows the bandwidths of blue and green lights emitted, allowing for better visualization of microvasculature and superficial mucosa. As haemoglobin absorbs blue light, hypervascular structures are more easily visualized, thus inflamed/early scarring may be more readily identified with this technology.

There is limited literature on the utility of this application in vocal fold scarring, but increasing evidence of the value of this technology in laryngeal dysplasia and malignancy[37].

Electroglottography

This technique traces the opening and the closing of the glottis performed by passing a low electrical current between the vocal folds during phonation. Vocal fold contact changes electrical impedance and these changes are shown plotted against time depicting the vocal fold cycle in wave-form. The tracings can be superimposed with the visual images. This may be helpful, as vocal fold scar can impair glottis closure.

Ultrasound

High-frequency miniaturized ultrasound transducers have been used in living tissue with near microscopic resolution[38]. Although there is limited literature on this modality evaluating human vocal folds for scar, it has potential as the echogenicity of tissue layers changes with the amount of collagen (hyperechoic) or elastin (hypoechoic). An ex-vivo proof-of-concept study has been performed demonstrating that with improved miniaturization of technology this technique can provide a view of the microstructure of the human vocal fold to aid in accurate diagnosis of scar and other pathologies[39].

Computerized tomography (CT) scanning

Using a spiral CT scanner, Abitbol *et al.*[40] acquired images of the larynx requiring only a 30-second exposure time. The scanner moves the subject continuously in a circle using volume acquisition imaging. Fundamental to the utility of the images is the post-processing analysis for 3D reconstruction, and the laryngologist should work with the radiologist at the workstation interpreting the images and changing contrast parameters if needed.

With further technological advancement, CT scanning may be used as an adjunct to diagnosis of vocal fold scarring. The main drawback at present is that volume rendering will create an artificially smooth surface of the endolaryngeal structures. As previously noted, the majority of scar will occur within the superficial layers of the vocal fold[5]. Radiation exposure is a further concern.

However the rapid acquisition of high-quality images for "virtual dissection[40]" of the larynx makes this an attractive potential modality for diagnosis.

Magnetic resonance imaging (MRI)

MRI is capable of multiplanar, high-resolution imaging that is often considered superior for soft tissue definition when compared to CT scan. In addition, patients are not exposed to radiation. However, movement artifacts can distort the images as the acquisition time is typically longer than CT scans. An ex-vivo study[41] using an 11.7 Tesla magnet has shown excellent images of the animal larynges can be obtained, thus detecting the presence of scar tissue. This should be corroborated with histological examination. MRI may be a useful tool in the future as technology advances.

References

1. Allen J. Cause of vocal cord scar. *Curr Opin Otolaryngol Head Neck Surg* 2010; 18:475–480
2. Fant G. *Acoustic Theory of Speech Production, With Calculations Based on X-ray Studies of Russian Articulations.* The Hague, the Netherlands: Mouton 1960.
3. Dikkers FG, Hulstaert CE, Oosterbaan JA, Cervera-Paz FJ. Ultrastructural changes of the basement membrane zone in benign lesions of the vocal folds. *Acta Otolaryngol* 1993; 113(1–2):98–101.
4. Gray SD, Hammond E, Hanson DF. Benign pathologic responses of the larynx. *Ann Otol Rhinol Laryngol* 1995; 104:13–18.
5. Rubin JS, Yanagisawa E. Benign laryngology through the eyes of the laryngologist. In: Rubin JS, Sataloff RT, Korovin G (Eds.) *Diagnosis and Treatment of Voice Disorders* 4 edn, San Diego, CA: Plural Publishing 2014.
6. Woo P. Diagnosis and management of postoperative dysphonia. In: Rubin JS, Sataloff RT, Korovin G, (Eds.) *Diagnosis and Treatment of Voice Disorders* 4 edn, San Diego, CA: Plural Publishing 2014.
7. Bouchayer M, Cornut G. Microsurgery for benign lesions of the vocal folds. *Ear Nose Throat J* 1988; 67:446–466.
8. Schwemmle C, Kreipe HH, Witte T, Ptok M. Bamboo nodes associated with mixed connective tissue disease as a cause of hoarseness. *Rheumatol Int* 2013; 33(3):777–81.
9. Ford CN, Inagi K, Khidir A, *et al.* Sulcus vocalis: a rational analytical approach to diagnosis and management. *Ann Otol Rhinol Laryngol* 1996; 105(3):189–00.
10. Jacobsen BH, Johnson A, Grywalski C, *et al.* The Voice Handicap Index (VHI): development and validation. *Am J Speech Lang Pathol* 1997; 6:66–70.
11. Rosen CA, Lee AS, Osborne J, *et al.* Development and validation of the Voice Handicap Index-10. *Laryngoscope* 2004; 114:1549–1556.

12. Friedrich G, Dikkers FG, Arens C, *et al.* Vocal fold scars: current concepts and future directions. Consensus report of the Phonosurgery Committee of the European Laryngological Society. *Eur Arch Otolaryngol* 2013; 270(9) 2491–2507.

13. Hirano M. Psycho-acoustic evaluation of voice: GRBAS scale for evaluating the hoarse voice. *Clinical Examination of the Voice* New York: Springer-Verlag 1981.

14. Mat Baki M, Wood G, Alston M, *et al.* Reliability of OperaVOX against Multidimensional Voice Program (MDVP). *Clin Otol* 2015; 40(1):22–28.

15. Mathieson L, Hirani S, Epstein R, *et al.* Laryngeal manual therapy: a preliminary study to examine its treatment effects in the management of muscle tension dysphonia. *J Voice* 2009; 23(3):353–366.

16. Korovin GS, Hughes O, Rubin JS. Introduction to the laboratory diagnosis of vocal disorders. In: Rubin JS, Sataloff RT, Korovin G (Eds.) *Diagnosis and Treatment of Voice Disorders* 4 edn, San Diego, CA: Plural Publishing 2014.

17. Eller R, Ginsburg M, Lurie D, *et al.* Flexible laryngoscopy: a comparison of fiber optic and distal chip technologies. Part 1: vocal fold masses. *J Voice* 2008; 22(6):746–750.

18. Bless DM, Hirano M, Feder RJ. Videostroboscopic evaluation of the larynx. *Ear Nose Throat J* 1987; 66:289–296.

19. Arens C, Remacle M. Scarred larynx. In: Remacle M, Eckel H (Eds.) *Surgery of the Larynx and Trachea*, Berlin: Springer Verlag 2010.

20. Tillmann B, Rudert H. Licht und elektronenmikroskopische untersuchungen zum reinkeodem. *HNO* 1982; 30:280–284.

21. Titze IR *Acoustic Voice Analysis: Summary Statement.* Iowa City, IA: National Center for Voice and Speech, 1994.

22. Baken RJ. *Clinical Measurement of Speech and Voice.* San Diego, CA: College-Hill Press 1987.

23. Dejonckere PH, Bradley P, Clemente P, *et al.* A basic protocol for functional assessment of voice pathology, especially for investigating the efficacy of (phonosurgical) treatments and evaluating new assessment techniques. *Eur Arch Otorhinolaryngol* 2001; 258:77–82.

24. Titze IR. *Workshop on Acoustic Voice Analysis: Summary Statement.* Iowa City IA: National Center for Voice and Speech 1995.

25. Hee Choi S, Zhang Y, Jiang JJ, *et al.* Nonlinear dynamic-based analysis of severe dysphonia in patients with vocal fold scar and sulcus vocalis. *J Voice* 2012; 26 (5):566–576.

26. Zhang Y, Jiang JJ, Wallace SM, Zhou L. Comparison of nonlinear dynamic methods and perturbation methods for voice analysis. *J Acoust Soc Am* 2005; 118:2551–2560.

27. Yu P, Garrel R, Nicollas R, *et al.* Objective voice analysis in dysphonic patients: new data including nonlinear measurements. *Folia Phoniatr Logop* 2007; 59:20–30.

28. Jiang JJ, Zhang Y, MacCallum J, *et al.* Objective acoustic analysis of pathological voices from patients with vocal nodules and polyps. *Folia Phoniatr Logop* 2009; 61:342–349.

29. Hillenbrand, J, Cleveland RA, Erickson, RL. Acoustic correlates of breathy vocal quality. *J Speech Hear Res* 1994; 37: 769–778.

30. Heman-Ackah Y, Sataloff R, Laureyns G, *et al*. Quantifying the cepstral peak prominence, a measure of dysphonia. *J Voice* 2014; 28:783–788.

31. Yumoto E. Aerodynamics, voice quality and laryngeal image analysis of normal and pathologic voices. *Curr Opin Otolaryngol Head Neck Surg* 2004; 12(3):166–173.

32. Chan RW, Titze IR. Dependence of phonation threshold pressure on vocal tract acoustics and vocal fold tissue mechanics. *J Acoust Soc Am* 2006; 119:2351–2362.

33. Woo P. Objective measures of laryngeal imaging: what have we learned since Dr. Paul Moore. *J Voice* 2014; 28:69–81.

34. Svec JG, Schutte HK. Videokymography: high-speed line scanning of vocal fold vibration. *J Voice*. 1996; 10(2):201–205.

35. Burns JA, Zeitels SM, Rox Anderson R, *et al*. Imaging the mucosa of the human vocal fold with optical coherence tomography. *Ann Otol Rhinol Laryngol* 2005; 114 (9):671–676.

36. Zeitels SM, Hillman RE, Desloge RB, *et al*. Phonomicrosurgery in singers and performing artists: treatment outcomes, management theories and future directions. *Ann Otol Rhinol Laryngol* Suppl 2002; 111(suppl 190):21–40.

37. Hawkshaw M, Sataloff J, Sataloff R. New concepts in vocal fold imaging – A review. *J Voice* 2013; 27(6):738–743

38. Che'rin E, Williams R, Needles A, *et al*. Ultrahigh frame rate retrospective ultrasound microimaging and blood flow visualization in mice in vivo. *Ultrasound Med Biol* 2006; 32:683–691.

39. Walsh CJ, Heaton JT, Kobler JB, *et al*. Imaging of the calf vocal fold with high-frequency ultrasound. *Laryngoscope* 2008; 118:1894–1899.

40. Abitbol J, Castro A, Gombergh R, Abitbol P. 3D Laryngeal CT scan for voice disorders: virtual endoscopy-virtual dissection. In: Rubin JS, Sataloff RT, Korovin G (Eds.) *Diagnosis and Treatment of Voice Disorders* 4ed, San Diego, CA: Plural Publishing 2014.

41. Herrera VLM, Viereck JC, Lopez-Guerra G, *et al*. 11.7 Tesla magnetic resonance microimaging of laryngeal tissue architecture. *Laryngoscope* 2009; 119: 2187–2194.

Section II

3

Voice therapy

Bridget Rose

Vocal impairment due to scar and its negative impact on patients are seen frequently by the speech-language pathologist. Many patients withdraw from social settings, resulting in diminishing interactions with friends and family. They also experience frustration because they must work harder to be understood as their volume, ease of phonation, and intelligibility may be impaired. Those who rely on their voices for a large part of their profession, such as coaches, school teachers, singing professionals, lecturers, supervisors, etc., may have to make major modifications in their occupational responsibilities. Many patients cease participating in activities that had given them much joy and fulfillment, such as avocational singing, due to their voice problems.

It has been noted in the literature and anecdotally that restoring functional voicing requires reducing inflammation, reducing/eliminating vocally traumatic behaviors, and providing new motor/mechanical learning patterns long after the vocal fold's functional epidermal barrier is restored[1-3]. Scar interferes with the smooth motion of the mucosal wave of the vocal folds due to the disruption of the vocal fold layers and impairment of vibration. This, in turn, leads to hoarseness, breathiness, strain, and fatigue[4]. Voice therapy is sufficient for some patients with scar. For others, pre-operative therapy should be encouraged by the voice team before surgical intervention, in addition to post-operative, restorative therapy, to allow for the best post-operative results.

There can be a myriad of difficulties encountered within speech/voice therapy treatment that arise from laryngeal pathologies, and scar is no exception. In fact, restoring a voice to its original, normal state is very rare[5]. The dysphonia, weakness, and resulting compensatory habits that patients accumulate create a challenge for the therapist. Frequently, vocal fold scar is not an isolated pathology, making therapy even more daunting. There is not a plethora of research about specific clinical therapies for scar as there are for some vocal fold pathologies. However, it is important that a voice clinician be familiar with basic research regarding origins and processes involved in wound repair and cellular activity[1-4]. Recent literature has referenced orthopedic rehabilitation of scar and the translational implications it might have for healing vocal fold scar tissue[1,6]. There is the suggestion that prolonged stretching, or the application of tension to fibrotic regions, can regain functional mobility at a wound site[1], and these findings may support the use of voice therapy in the treatment of vocal fold scar. This background should be helpful in setting individual goals and providing realistic expectations for patients.

This chapter provides suggestions regarding initial evaluation, as well as follow up therapy techniques (both indirect and direct) that are intended to be implemented both pre- and post-surgically.

Initial evaluation

Before the actual speech/voice therapy begins, there should be a thorough discussion of the diagnosis and plan of care with the treating otolaryngologist. A complete history is done by the treating speech pathologist who is an experienced and professionally licensed clinician, preferably with special training or a background in voice. This requires knowing the onset of events and how the patient has acclimated to symptoms and any ramifications of this. In addition to the initial "why are you here today" questions, other enquiries should include daily voice use at work, socially, and at home. Specific symptoms should be identified. Many patients with scar complain of vocal fatigue, pitch breaks, inability to control voice, and dysphonia/hoarseness. Identifying the patient's specific goals and determining if they are realistic are important to successful therapy.

Ideally, acoustic and aerodynamic measurements are completed before diagnostic trials. Objective voice data are invaluable pre- and post-treatment (and periodically throughout) to observe/evaluate therapy effectiveness[5,7]. Measurements are taken first to avoid any bias from trial therapy during the initial session. Acoustic and aerodynamic testing should be performed in a sound isolated room, when possible. Recordings of sustained phonemes and running speech allow for quantifying perturbation measures such as fundamental frequency (Hz), Noise-to-harmonic ratio, S/Z ratios, maximum phonation time, jitter and shimmer, and average sound pressure levels (dB). At our voice clinic we perform most of these tests using the *Multi-Dimensional Voice Parameters®* (MDVP) (KayPentax, PENTAX Medical, Montvale, NJ) instrumentation programs. Aerodynamic measurements are valuable and Cepstral peak prominence is also a useful measure of dysphonia[8]. A spirometer may also be used as a quick screening tool to determine whether pulmonary function referral and follow up are needed. If one does not have more sophisticated instrumentation, such as the Computerized Speech Lab (CSL) or Phonatory Aerodynamic System (PAS) by KayPentax, then measument of S/Z ratio, maximum phonation time, and pitch range can be recorded with a stopwatch and keyboard (or keyboard phone app) and used as pre-post therapy references.

The S/Z ratio often is used to help assess glottic closure. It tests for hyper and hypo function and individual vocal efficiency. There are normative ranges for genders and age, with the mean being 1.0 for both genders in adults. To find the ratio, maximum phonation time on /s/ is divided by maximum phonation time on /z/. A reduced S/Z ratio is associated with hypofunction and elevated S/Z ratio is associated with hyperfunction. Hyperfunction is often found in patients with scar. Maximum phonation time (MPT) measures the duration of extended phonation (average of three trials) on the vowel /α/ on a comfortable pitch provided by a keyboard, pitch pipe, or other instrument. Pitch range from highest pitch (Hz) to lowest pitch (hz) also can be assessed on MDVP or keyboard.

There are several validated instruments that help standardize perceptions of voice[9-12]. The VRQOL (Voice Related Quality of Life) and VHI-10 (Vocal Handicap Index-ten questions), for example, are self-perception questionnaires completed by patients. The GRBAS scale (Grade, Roughness, Breathiness, Asthenia and Strain) and the CAPE-V (Consensus Auditory Perceptual Evaluation of Voice) are completed by clinicians. These all add value to the clinician's assessment and enhanced understanding of patients' perceptions of their vocal problems. These may be used again post-operatively and after a course of therapy to document progress[9-12].

Ideally, the speech-language pathologist's initial evaluation session should include a brief review of anatomy of the larynx/voice, clinician auditory assessment of patient's dysphonia, observations of postural alignment and breath management, and therapeutic trials utilizing appropriate vocal exercises. Diagnostic trial therapy during the initial evaluation allows the clinician to observe the patient's facility and comprehension of tasks and assess likelihood of future compliance.

Indirect therapy

Vocal hygiene is considered an indirect means of therapy and encompasses many topics including environmental factors, hydration, potential dietary modifications, medication use, and vocal misuse. Clinicians can help identify potential negative behaviors and provide alternative suggestions to modify or eliminate them[5,12]. Greater awareness of these topics and subsequent behavioral modifications can contribute to improved therapy outcomes. Specific items to consider are appropriate hydration and avoidance of irritants, as well as elimination of potentially drying agents (or mucus-thickening agents) such as antihistamines. Injurious behaviors such as throat clearing, coughing, and yelling should be identified. Strategies to minimize or eliminate these behaviors should be implemented[13]. Techniques including silent cough, hard swallowing, and nasal breathing can be introduced. Amplification can assist patients who need to project their voices. Control of laryngopharyngeal reflux with diet and lifestyle modification can be discussed in addition to medical management by the physician, but physician advice can be reinforced by the speech-language pathologist[13-17].

Amplification

Amplification devices allow patients an excellent opportunity to reduce strain and current or potential vocal trauma in work and social settings. Amplification may improve ease and comfort during phonation, and reduce fatigue without the patient compromising newly acquired voicing techniques or engaging in repetitive, acute phonotrauma. It is important to emphasize to the patient that the amplification device is a means of vocal preservation.

Direct voice therapy

One of the biggest obstacles to patients in therapy is a lack of awareness of the quality of his/her voice production. As therapists, one of our main goals is to cultivate that awareness; increasing patient self-perception beyond that of how the voice "sounds" and moving towards what the patient "feels" during speech[3]. Patients should be engaged in the various "placements" of vibratory sensations during speech. As a consequence, they often become aware of the presence of unnecessary tension in the tongue, neck, and jaw and the need for a more appropriate, usually slower, rate of speech, efficient use of breath, and improved anterior tone focus.

During therapy, coordination of the subsystems that create efficient vocal production is emphasized, specifically the respiratory, phonatory, and resonance systems. The exercises discussed here are intended to create a more efficient and effective symbiosis of these functions, including reducing glottic insufficiency and, most importantly, improving the scar-compromised mucosal wave.

Many patients have a concomitant diagnosis of muscle tension dysphonia. It may be difficult to determine whether this is compensation for pathology or preceded (or caused) by the pathology. Reducing laryngeal and extralaryngeal tension to achieve a more harmonious working of the laryngeal mechanism must be addressed. Neutral postural alignment may reduce head and neck strain and prevent the larynx from rising unnecessarily. Laryngeal massage addresses intrinsic and extrinsic laryngeal muscular tension. Abdominal breathing tasks aid in effective and efficient airflow during phonation, and stretch and massage reduce facial musculature and tongue tension. A series of stretches, massage, and relaxation tasks that can be done by the patient at home are discussed briefly.

If a clinician is not familiar with laryngeal palpation and circumlaryngeal massage, training from a knowledgeable speech-language pathologist and/or laryngologist is essential. Laryngeal massage can be taught to patients in full or in modification. Many patients who have dysphonia related to scar can experience reduced tension and strain in the neck musculature and a sensation of "open feeling" in the throat accompanied by an ease of vocal production immediately following massage. Audibly, voices may sound more clear and less rough[7,18].

Tongue tension releasing tasks include stretches in isolation and tongue-out speech. Patients may hold gentle stretches lasting anywhere from 10–20 seconds while protruding the tongue on the bottom lip. Having the patient hold his/her tongue in position outside the mouth can be helpful to facilitate the stability of placement and stretch. As the patient speaks with the tongue out, he/she can use rote phrases (e.g. days of the week, counting 1–10). The patient may manually hold his/her tongue out gently, if the tendency is to pull it backwards into mouth during phonation. This is done several times to "ensure tongue muscles have stretched and relaxed" to prevent further immediate hyperfunction[19]. Many patients who present with tongue base tension find immediate carry-over of improved ease of speech after several repetitions of this task.

Stretch and relaxation tasks involve a series of head and neck stretches that often help decrease strain and improve the comfortable range of motion. These should be modified or eliminated if the patient has bodily limitations such as of cervical arthritis, neck injuries, or shoulder injuries[15]. Suggestions include, but are not limited to, facial massage focusing on temporal and masseter musculature and head rolls gently from shoulder to shoulder while utilizing cyclical continuous breathing. The patient may release air on an aspirate consonant so as to avoid any laryngeal "lock" or pressure during the stretch. The patient may also utilize a slight chin elevation for a gentle stretch during air release; a gentle stretch of the neck (ear to shoulder) right and left; and a neck turn gently toward/ slightly over each shoulder being aware of the stretch in the neck musculature bilaterally. Shoulder rolls with the chin to chest to avoid compression of the back of the neck, as well as posterior neck self-massage, may be completed.

Clinicians should observe a patient's posture with the goal of neutral head and neck alignment and balance. Neutral postural alignment may allow for more efficient voicing[15,19]. Habitual issues, such as chin and head jutting/lifting up or forward, may be associated with laryngeal rise and tension and back of neck/ cervical compression. Standing with weight either only on the balls of the feet or heels may contribute to undue strain and uncoordinated breathing. Use of a mirror for full body observation may help patients reorganize negative postural compensatory habits.

Efficient breath use

Sustainable, functional voice use requires efficient breathing/breath support. Abdominal breathing tasks help improve patients' awareness of unnecessary force, underuse of support musculature or paradoxical abdominal movements. Observation of patient breathing habits may reveal undesirable patterns. Does the patient demonstrate tension in the shoulders or chest? Does he/she demonstrate a thoracic or clavicular breathing pattern? If so, is there habitual breath holding? The larynx may compensate with excessively forceful glottic closure in these positions. It may not be necessary to spend a lot of time on breathing patterns beyond basics unless a patient struggles with breathing-related problems. Many tasks, such as semi-occluded lip trills and tongue-out trills, may facilitate spontaneous breath coordination and awareness. Visual observation with mirrors is recommended, as is tactile/hands on positioning, for increased body awareness. Patient observations of their body movements during a breath cycle may include chest movement (up/down), upper and lower abdominal movement, and back expansion. Something as simple as taking a gentle breath in through a drinking straw with a cue to observe abdominal movement can increase awareness and help to change a clavicular breathing pattern into an abdominal/diaphragmatic one. Simple breathing tasks for improved awareness and facility include comfortable, cyclical breathing exercises. Visualization of a continuous cycle (circle) of breath with no halts or pauses in between should be encouraged. Patients should be cued to inhale comfortably through the nose and exhale on unvoiced phonemes /s/, /f/ and "sh." During inhalation, shoulders should remain relaxed and abdominal muscles should release gently. Exhalation is not forceful. Toward the end of exhalation, abdominal muscles should be allowed to move slightly in towards the spine and up in order to support airflow. However, excessive abdominal excursion may impair support. Greater awareness of changes in body movement and support often occurs with practice in different positions. While lying on the floor with a hand on the abdomen, a release of upper body tension and increased abdominal movement often are observed. This also may be noted while sitting in a chair with chest "open" and sternum gently raised. Breathing tasks can then translate into a hierarchy of speech tasks as deemed necessary. A relative, overall feeling of calm and relaxation is an ideal start to sessions.

Yawn–sigh–hum

Initiating a yawn is one way to release or relax tense laryngeal and extralaryngeal musculature, which frequently manifests as a higher-than-necessary laryngeal position. Patients are asked to yawn, and anything to help stimulate that, including clinician demonstration, can facilitate this act[14]. Ideal yawn posture gently increases oropharyngeal space. The tongue tip should be relaxed behind the bottom front teeth. The patient transitions using a breathy sigh on exhalation. Exhalation can move to voicing with the word "hum," initiated with the "yawn-sigh," and ending with closed lips on an anterior tone focused /m/ placement.

There should be a resonant, vibratory sensation on the lips, alveolar ridge, and in the facial bones. This is often an excellent cue to segue to semi-occluded tasks such as the lip trill or resonant voicing on the nasal consonant /m/.

Semi-occluded vocal tract tasks

Standard semi-occluded vocal tract (SOVT) exercises used in therapy that facilitate increased vocal fold amplitude, increased sound pressure levels, and increased anterior tone focus/resonance may include lip trills (bubbles or rolled /r/), tongue out trills ("raspberries"), resonant voicing tasks (sustained nasals /m/, /n/), and straw phonation. These may be beneficial for increased tone focus without instigating further vocal trauma, strain, or force[7,14,20-22]. SOVT exercises facilitate decreased vocal effort during phonation, increased patient awareness of anterior tone focus, and increased clarity of tone; and it allows for improved awareness of breath/respiratory support and facilitates carry-over into speech.

Lip trills and tongue trills are often an appropriate first voiced task for patients as they work towards an increased awareness of vocal system coordination. Benefits include decreased laryngeal strain, anterior facial tone focus, and improved abdominal support[12,14,15,19]. The patient initiates the task with an unvoiced trill/bubble and transitions to a voiced trill while experimenting with a comfortable pitch range. Finger tips near the corners of the mouth during the lip buzz may facilitate increased anterior tone sensation and reduce neck strain. Pitch glides on gradually increased ascending and descending patterns on either lip or tongue trills should be included as part of a patient's daily vocal warm-up and cool-down routine.

Straw phonation tasks can be practiced with a thin coffee stirring straw or a drinking straw that is slightly larger in diameter. These exercises have been shown to reduce vocal fold impact and result in an improved sensation of facial resonance and unforced improvements in vocal clarity, volume, and mucosal wave[20-22]. Straw phonation on ascending and descending glides using solitary vowels on /i/, /u/, and /ɑ/ may be utilized with and without water resistance. Nasal air emission should be avoided. Simple instructions include having the patient place the tip of a plastic straw in the mouth and gently blow air through on a phoneme. Cues for more released cheek musculature (slightly puffy) may allow for further decrease in noticeable jaw tension. Cues for a secure lip seal without lip tension/pressing encourage an increased anterior tone focused "buzz-like" sensation. The author allows patients to begin with descending glides from a comfortable pitch, which are provided by clinician or a keyboard pitch cue. The patient then glides gently from a lower comfortable pitch to higher, being careful to avoid pitch extremes at this point, keeping throat/upper body as relaxed as possible, with awareness of gently engaged abdominal support. He/she continues with pitch glides allowing for the "buzz" sensation on the lips and tip of the straw. Therapy advances by having the patient speak and/or sing a phrase or token melody into the straw and then without the straw. These tasks appear to be very efficient in helping carry over improved ease of phonation and anterior tone quality in speech[20-22].

Flow phonation tasks with water-filled cups can be an effective tool for many patients demonstrating all levels (mild–severe) of dysphonia due to scar. These exercises allow for increased subglottic airflow without excess neck and laryngeal strain[12]. They may facilitate awareness of airflow (visual), reduced vocal fold force, and reduced strain during phonation. Patients often comment that the visual aspect allows for greater understanding of respiratory and phonatory coordination. Cup bubble facilitator exercises are simply speech into water without a straw. A patient brings a cup of water to his/her lips (approximately 1/3 to 1/4 cup of water is adequate) and begins to gently blow air, or unvoiced bubbles. They then add voice with ease of onset, which allows awareness of airflow (and even abdominal support changes) without worrying about context. This segues to voicing with a solitary vowel (e.g. /u/, /ou/, /i/), and phonation is sustained for several seconds. Patients can progress to descending pitch glides quickly on the same sounds. The number of trials (e.g. 5–10x) may be alternated, and the vowels may be varied[12]. The exercise continues to speech in a hierarchy of tasks starting with words and progressing to phrase and sentence levels. Choosing a word that begins with "w" facilitates the glide and continuation of /u/ vowel. The patient maintains the tone on the vowel and voices the word of choice. Phonation can be alternated with the water and then without in order to allow for sensation of carry-over of the improved resonant placement and ease of phonation. The tasks advance to short phrase (e.g. "why not") and sentence levels (e.g. "Where are you going?").

Resonant voice therapy (RVT)

Resonant voicing techniques are utilized for those with vocal fold scar as a means to encourage increased mucosal wave vibration, anterior tone focus, and easy phonation. During voicing, vocal fold contact forces are minimized, so the low impact element of this therapy is thought to help prevent further injury and allow for reduced stiffness of scar tissue[6]. It involves large amplitude, low impact, stress vocal fold oscillations that may greatly help reduce mechanical stress on the vocal folds[1,6]. The gentle vocal fold adduction/contact increases vocal resonance vibrations perceived on the alveolar ridge, lips, tongue, nasal bridge, and facial bones[3,7,12]. Many speech-language pathologists have had some kind of introduction to resonant voice therapy, but a useful formal protocol, Lessac-Madsen Resonant Voice Therapy (LMRVT), was developed by Katherine Verdolini-Abbott[3,12]. It includes vocal hygiene, stretching and breathing maneuvers, alternating voiced and voiceless phonemes, forward tone focus, and experience in sensation of anterior tone focus. It proceeds with a hierarchy of steps utilizing single consonant–vowel (CV) and consonant–vowel–consonant–vowel (CVCV) combinations within speech and chant speech. This progresses from word to phrase, to paragraph reading to controlled conversation, and finally to conversational speech.

Vocal function exercises

The vocal function exercise (VFEs) protocol mentioned here was described by Dr. Joseph Stemple, CCC-SLP, and may be introduced to patients in tandem with other voicing techniques. VFEs are lower impact tasks designed to improve the balance of the laryngeal mechanism by increasing the stamina, strength, and flexibility of the vocal folds while reducing/eliminating laryngeal and extralaryngeal tension[7]. The timing of implementing these tasks should be influenced by the progress of the patient. If a patient has a fairly good grasp of SOVT tasks, is reasonably comfortable with abdominal breathing habits, and has made progress with reducing/eliminating compensatory tensions, VFEs can be an excellent way to improve glottic insufficiency. The clinician may start with the program as a whole, or incorporate the pitch glide tasks initially and graduate to the whole protocol. These exercises consist of four specific tasks to be completed twice daily, and many patients have found this structured practice easy to fit into busy schedules. It requires a stopwatch/ timer, keyboard or keyboard phone app, or pitch pipe, and a means to document daily practice results. Tasks include: maximum phonation times on the vowel /i/, ascending and descending pitch glides with focus on a forward "buzzy–oo" or "whistle tone-like" sensation, and sustained phonation on the vowel /u/ on five distinct pitches which are to be agreed upon by the clinician and patient[7,12]. It is important to remember that VFE tasks are executed without forced or pressed phonation at softer vocal levels. Standard protocol lasts for approximately 6–8 weeks and is tapered off or modified for continuous maintenance according to individual patient needs.

Post-operative therapy

Pre-operative therapy for vocal fold scar is an invaluable asset for many patients post-peratively, as it allows for greater facility, awareness, and coordination of new mechanical and behavioral patterns. Before a surgical procedure, the patient should be comfortable with newly acquired skills in order to facilitate optimal healing and return to atraumatic voice use. Patient facility and comprehension of these techniques during pre-operative therapy may greatly improve post-operative phonation due to newly learned awareness of vocal placement or "sensations" and ingrained muscle memory. While there is a variety of immediate post-operative voice therapy protocols, most surgeons prescribe a period of complete and/or modified voice rest. Clinicians should review and reinforce the need for compliance, including vocal use restrictions, vocal hygiene, dietary modifications if any, reflux treatments, and physical activities as specified by the physician. Post-operative voice recovery may span approximately 1–6 weeks. Therefore, restrictions may include limited phone use, avoidance of coughing, throat clearing, heavy lifting, smoking, and use of anticoagulants as specified by the surgeon. After the patient is cleared for voice use, a recovery protocol is used. Many specialized voice clinics will employ a specific approach to re-introducing voice use post-operatively. During this period, the therapist continues instruction with an alternative voicing and vocal rest protocol and treatment at least weekly when possible. Controlled phonation alternating with voice rest helps healing more readily than spontaneous, unmonitored/untrained post-operative phonation[23]. Weekly, or more frequent, post-operative therapy visits are initially short, 30 minute durations (or less), and usually return to standard 50-minute therapy sessions after 2 weeks. At any time, the speech-language pathologist may modify/change the structure of the voiced/unvoiced protocol if the patient experiences fatigue, dysphonia, or pain during recovery. Other voice team members should be informed if this is necessary.

Patients should have a practice routine that is tailored and proven effective for them and is adaptable to their daily schedules. Practicing anywhere from 3–5 times daily at 5-–15 minute intervals may be sufficient. The frequency and duration can increase as progress increases and must be individualized. Every patient should have an initial vocal warm-up plan that takes only 10–15 minutes as well as a vocal cool-down plan, both of which are learned pre-operatively and re-introduced after surgery.

The treating speech-language pathologist will continue with the hierarchy of tasks as the patient's functional voice use improves. If progress halts or plateaus, the patient should be referred for early re-evaluation to the physician. If the progress plateaus and the patient is pleased and/or has accepted his/her vocal condition, discharge is appropriate. However, periodic follow up is prudent, and patients are asked to return six weeks after "discharge" to evaluate carry-over. Even after a course of voice therapy, which may range from 6–12 sessions and sometimes more, the vocal fold tissue repair can continue up to 12 months post-operatively[1,6]. Continued maintenance and re-evaluation with the voice team is highly encouraged, because wound healing and tissue repair continue after injury.[1] Thorough understanding of the limitations of the scar pathology, healing/recovery time frames, and variability of impairment from patient to patient, will result in appropriate therapy tailored to individual patients. There are no guarantees with treatment of vocal fold scar, but it is essential to know the patient's functional goals, motivation, and to encourage compliance in order to achieve most successful outcome.

References

1. Branski RC, Verdolini K, Sandulache V, *et al*. Vocal fold wound healing: a review for clinicians. *J Voice* 2006 Sep; 20(3):432–442.
2. Hansen JK, Thibeault, S. Current understanding and review of the literature: Vocal fold scarring. *J Voice* 2006; 20(1):110–120.
3. Verdolini K. *Resonant Voice Therapy: National Center for Voice and Speech's Guide to Vocology*. Iowa City, IA: National Center for Voice and Speech; 1998; 34–35.
4. Heman-Ackah YD, Sataloff RT, Hawkshaw MJ. *The Voice: A Medical Guide for Achieving and Maintaining a Healthy Voice*. Narberth, PA: Science and Medicine, Inc. 2013.
5. Rubin JS, Sataloff RT, Korovin GS (Eds.). *Diagnosis and Treatment of Voice Disorders* 4 edn, San Diego, CA: Plural Publishing 2014; Ch. 24,39,40.
6. Verdolini Abbott K, Li NYK, Branski RC, *et al*. Vocal exercise may attenuate acute vocal fold inflammation. *J Voice* 2012 Nov; 26(6):814.e1–13.
7. Stemple JC, Glaze LE, Gerdeman Kalben B. *Clinical Voice Pathology: Theory and Management* 3 edn. San Diego, CA: Singular Publishing Group 2000; Ch. 6, 179–254.Ch. 7, 335–340.
8. Heman-Ackah YD, Sataloff RT, Laureyns G, *et al*. Quantifying the cepstral peak prominence, a measure of dysphonia. *J Voice* 2014 Nov; 28(6):783–788.

9. Da Costa de Ceballos AG, Carvalho FM, de Araújo TM, Farias Borges dos Reis EJ. Diagnostic validity of Voice Handicap Index-10 (VHI-10) compared with perceptive-auditory and acoustic speech pathology evaluations of the voice. *J Voice* 2010 Nov; 24(6):715–718.

10. Portone CR, Hapner ER, McGregor L, *et al*. Correlation of the Voice Handicap Index (VHI) and the Voice-Related Quality of Life Measure (V-RQOL). *J Voice* 2007 Nov; 21(6):723–727.

11. Zraick RI, Kempster GB, Connor NP, *et al*. Establishing validity of the Consensus Auditory-Perceptual Evaluation of Voice (CAPE-V) *Am J Speech Lang Pathol* 2011; 20:14–22.

12. Stemple J, Hapner, ER. *Voice Therapy: Clinical Case Studies* 4 edn. San Diego, CA: Plural Publishing, Inc. 2014;Ch.1, 1–10, Ch.3, 49, 111–115, 142–157, Ch.7, 443–452.

13. Zwitman, Calcaterra T. The "silent cough" method for vocal hyperfunction. *J Speech Hear Disord* 1973; 38:119–125.

14. Colton RH, Casper JK, Leonard R. *Understanding Voice Problems: A Physiological Perspective for Diagnosis and Treatment* 4 edn. Philadelphia, PA: Lippincott, Williams and Wilkins 2011; 10, 14.

15. Sataloff RT. *Vocal Health and Pedagogy*. San Diego, CA: Singular Publishing Group 1998.

16. Aviv J. *Killing Me Softly from Inside*. New York: CNB Productions, LLC. 2012.

17. Koufman J., *Dropping Acid: The Reflux Diet Cookbook and Cure*. Elmwood Park, NJ: G&H Soho, Inc. 2010.

18. Roy N, Bless DM, Heisey D, Ford CN. Manual circumlaryngeal therapy for functional dysphonia: An evaluation of short and long term treatment outcomes. *J Voice* 1997; 3:321–331.

19. Sataloff, RT. *The Professional Voice: Part II. The Science and Art of Clinical Care*. New York, NY: Raven Press 1991; 68. F.

20. Guzman M, Laukkanen AM, Krupa P, *et al*. Vocal tract and glottal function during and after vocal exercising with resonance tube and straw. *J Voice* 2013; 27(4):523. e19–523e34.

21. Guzman M, Higueras D, Fincheira C, *et al*. Immediate acoustic effects of straw phonation exercises in subjects with dysphonic voices. *Logoped Phoniatr Vocol* 2013; 38:35–45.

22. Titze I. Voice training and therapy with a semi occluded vocal tract: rational and scientific underpinnings. *J Speech Lang Hear Res* 2006; 49:448–459.

23. Ishikawa K, Thibeault S. Voice rest versus exercise: A review of the literature. *J Voice* 2010; 24(4):379–387.

4

Medical management

Scott Hardison

Scarring causes disruption of the unique architecture of the vocal fold, inhibiting the formation and propagation of the mucosal wave necessary for normal voice production. The sequence of scar formation is well described as it relates to the dermis, and these mechanisms typically are applied to the formation of vocal fold scar, although this is not as well studied (Figure 4.1). By targeting various points in this sequence of events, it might be possible to prevent or even reverse formation of scar tissue within the layers of the vocal fold. This has been the focus of a number of studies in recent years and holds considerable promise in helping to preserve and restore the voices of patients with vocal fold scar. Beyond medical management of laryngopharyngeal reflux, allergies, and other disorders that can cause inflammation of the larynx, there are three medications directed at the prevention and treatment of vocal fold scar. These include corticosteroids, Mitomycin C, and 5-Fluorouracil.

Corticosteroids

The anti-inflammatory effects of steroids are due largely to their regulation of the production of cytokines and other inflammatory mediators. This typically occurs at the genetic and cellular level, with steroids inhibiting certain pro-inflammatory genes responsible for encoding cytokines in macrophages, mast cells and lymphocytes[1]. This, in turn, prevents activation of lymphocytes. Simultaneously, these same steroids activate other genes that govern the production of anti-inflammatory factors, including enzymes that stabilize

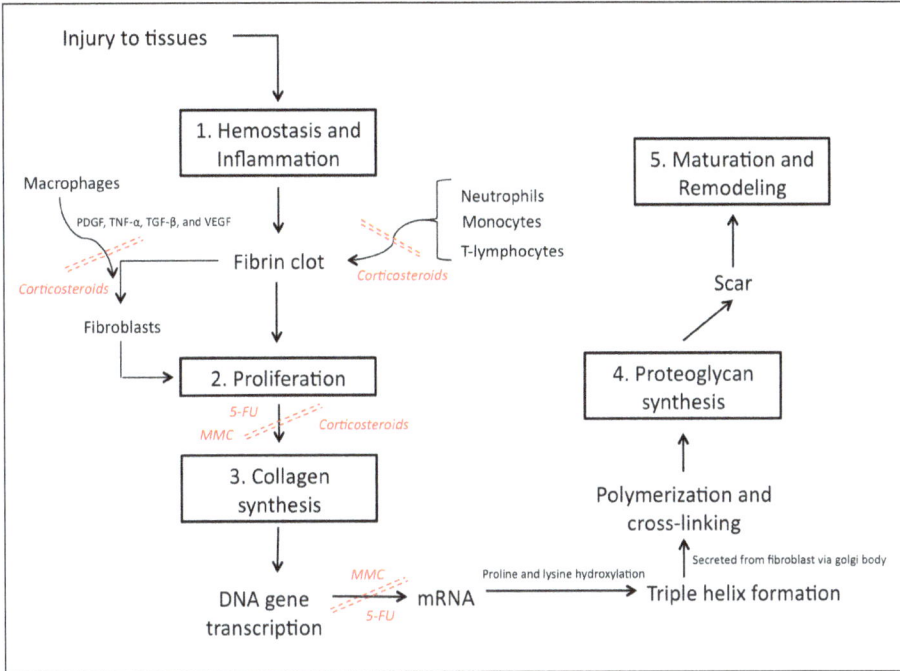

Figure 4.1 Mechanism for scar formation. Red dotted lines represent points in the cycle at which the various medications being discussed act on scar formation. MMC = Mitomycin C, 5-FU = 5-fluorouracil.

lysosomes and prevent release of chemotactic and vasoactive substances[1]. Notably, steroids have also been found to inhibit fibroblast proliferation, which offers yet another mechanism by which they may be used to prevent scarring[2] (Figure 4.1).

Despite their many therapeutic benefits, steroids have a number of well-documented side effects when used systemically. These include immunosuppression, insomnia, fluid retention, weight gain, osteoporosis, and fluctuations in blood glucose. For this reason, local administration of steroids is often appropriate when treating laryngeal conditions.

Clinical use

Steroids typically are used in laryngeal surgery in the form of injection. These injections are commonly performed in the operating room as part of microsuspension direct laryngoscopy (MDL) and may be performed prophylactically or therapeutically. Additionally, steroid injection can be accomplished in the office via a per-oral or per-cutaneous technique as described in other chapters.

Prophylactic steroid injections are employed by many laryngologists to prevent scarring after laryngeal microsurgery. This typically involves injection of the steroids into the superficial lamina propria, theoretically preventing scarring. This method was studied in an animal model by Campagnolo et al[3]. In this study, the investigators performed bilateral microflap surgeries on 12 rabbits. Dexamethasone was injected into the left true vocal fold of each rabbit, and no steroid treatment was performed on the right true vocal fold (serving as a control). Animals were sacrificed at 3 and 7 days. Immune response and scar deposition were quantified using special stains, revealing no significant difference in immune response but a significantly lower rate of collagen deposition in the steroid-treated vocal folds ($p = 0.002$).

Therapeutic steroid injections also have been the subject of investigation for the treatment of vocal fold scar. Mortensen and Woo investigated the performance of laryngeal steroid injections in an office setting[4]. In this retrospective review, 34 patients with postoperative vocal fold scarring, nodules, or sarcoidosis/granuloma were selected to undergo injection of methylprednisolone in the office per-oral. Statistically significant improvement was seen in voice grade, amplitude, and mucosal wave. No complications were noted, and the procedure was generally tolerated well by the patients involved in the study. A prospective multicenter study was conducted in 2011 by Woo et al. to evaluate percutaneous vocal fold injections in the treatment of benign lesions, including vocal fold scar[5]. A total of 115 patients who had refused general anesthesia and showed no response to voice therapy underwent these injections in an office setting. Most subjective and objective parameters demonstrated statistically significant improvement at the first and third months after injection, with no severe complications noted.

When contemplating the use of injectable steroids, whether for prophylactic or therapeutic treatments, the selection of the most appropriate steroid is important. Corticosteroids vary based on the strength and duration of action of their glucocorticoid groups. Table 4.1 summarizes the most common corticosteroids and their relative strengths[1].

Table 4.1 Glucocorticoid equivalence, systemic administration. Adapted from Campagnolo *et al*[2].

Drug	Dose equivalent (mg)	Biologic half-life (hours)
Betamethasone	1	24-72
Dexamethasone	1.5	24-72
Methyl-prednisolone	8	18-36
Triamcinolone	8	18-36
Prednisone	10	18-36
Prednisolone	10	18-36
Hydrocortisone	40	8-12
Cortisone	50	8-12

With local use of steroids, a longer biologic half-life confers a distinct advantage, as dosing will typically occur only once. Additionally, injection into a confined space such as the superficial lamina propria limits the volume of the injection, favoring steroids with higher anti-inflammatory strength. Another consideration is the preparation of the drug itself. Some steroids that are used routinely in local injections elsewhere in the body, most notably triamcinolone (Kenalog®, Bristol-Myers Squibb Company, Princeton, NJ), are prepared as a suspension and have a tendency to crystallize in the tissue, thus leaving behind a residue. This is not suitable in the superficial lamina propria, where the deposition of any material may have a negative effect on propagation of the mucosal wave[6]. With these criteria in mind, dexamethasone (Decadron®, Merck and Co., Inc., Whitehouse Station, NJ) has emerged as a well-suited choice, having excellent strength and a long half-life, coupled with its ability to dissolve fully within the tissues.

Mitomycin C

Mitomycin C (MMC) is a naturally derived antibiotic and chemotherapeutic agent. It is isolated from *Streptomyces caespitosus*, a gram negative bacterium[7]. MMC is an alkylating agent, meaning that it cross-links DNA and prevents the double strands from separating during replication. This effectively inhibits mitosis in the cells that the drug comes into contact with. MMC has an effect on fibroblast proliferation[8-12]. A recent study by Li *et al.* showed this effect to be dose-dependent when MMC was tested on colonies of fibroblasts[7] (Figure 4.1).

In addition to inhibiting DNA replication, MMC also has the ability to bind to promoter sites on genes, thus preventing protein synthesis[13]. In fibroblasts, this mechanism prevents the transcription of the genes encoding collagen (Figure 4.1). This inhibition of collagen synthesis, in addition to the decrease in fibroblast proliferation caused by MMC, leads to decreased scar formation.

Despite the clear benefits of MMC in decreasing scarring, its nonspecific effects may lead to apoptosis and inhibit protein synthesis in other cell populations[14]. This has been studied in airway use, with some studies showing fibrinous debris obstructing the airway[15], significant eschar in a rabbit model[16], and even a case of laryngeal cancer within 3 years of treatment[17]. MMC also may damage normal vocal fold tissue with which it comes in contact[18]. Despite these reported complications, local administration of MMC limits its affects to that immediate area and avoids systemic toxicity.

Clinical use

MMC treatment of laryngeal scar is typically performed prophylactically. In one study by Pereira *et al.*19, investigators performed direct laryngoscopy on a swine model. The animals were divided into three groups, with the control group undergoing topical application of normal saline via a pledget applied to uninjured vocal folds. The two treatment groups received separate doses of MMC by application of pledgets. The animals were sacrificed at 30 days, the final histology failing to reveal a noticeable difference in submucosal collagen deposition. This study has limitations including those of a small sample size and uninjured vocal folds that would not have been actively producing scar tissue. It also was performed on an animal model that may not mimic human vocal fold response.

Studies performed in humans, however, have shown more promise. A prospective controlled trial performed by Fawaz *et al.* studied a group of 25 patients undergoing posterior transverse laser cordotomy for treatment of bilateral true vocal fold paralysis[20]. The patients were divided into two groups, with one undergoing surgery alone and the other group undergoing both surgery and topical application of MMC. The patients in the treatment arm of the study demonstrated significantly less granulation tissue on the true vocal folds, as well as significantly less subjective dyspnea.

The majority of practitioners performing studies on this medication administer the treatment topically. This may be performed during direct laryngoscopy, with most reports describing a single application of MMC, typically at a concentration of 0.4 mg/mL, with the medication-soaked pledget remaining in place for a brief period of time (2–4 minutes). The site is commonly washed with topical lidocaine, and all excess irrigant is removed. Overall, results within the literature have been promising, but no firm protocols or guidelines currently exist for the use of this medication in the larynx.

5-fluorouracil

The drug 5-fluorouracil (5-FU) is a pyrimidine analog that has a broad spectrum of clinical applications. Its uses range from chemotherapy for head and neck cancer and breast cancer to the topical treatment of actinic keratosis and basal cell carcinoma of the skin (Efudex®, Valeant Pharmaceuticals International, Inc., Laval Quebec, Canada). Since the late 1980s, the drug also has seen use as an intralesional injection for hypertrophic scars and keloids[21].

Once inside cells, 5-FU acts by a few different mechanisms. First, it has the ability to bind the enzyme thymidylate synthase, which results in decreased production of thymidine, thus blocking DNA replication[22]. Second, the drug is able to integrate into DNA that is being replicated, acting as a mutagen that incorporates guanine into the wrong location on various genes[22]. This can have dramatic downstream effects, including inhibited production of proteins or apoptosis. These mechanisms all contribute to the effects of this drug on fibroblast proliferation and collagen production.

Systemic use of this medication may lead to many of the toxicities associated with other forms of chemotherapeutic agents, such as pancytopenia, anemia, stomatitis and cardiac injury[23]. Local use, however, has fewer associated side effects. These typically consist of local irritation and burning, although there is some question as to whether 5-FU could cause local teratogenicity[23].

Clinical use

Recent studies of the use of 5-fluorouracil (5-FU) have centered on topical administration of the drug. One interesting study performed by Baptistella *et al.*[24] compared both MMC and 5-FU to a control in pigs that had undergone CO_2 laser partial excision of the vocal folds. In the two treatment groups, the left fold was used as a control and the right fold had a pledget soaked with the respective drug applied for 3 minutes. The control group underwent surgery only, and both vocal folds were left untreated. When the animals were euthanized at 30 days, the MMC and 5-FU animals were found to have significantly less collagen deposition as compared to the control animals. Interestingly, there was no significant difference noted between the MMC and 5-FU groups, suggesting similar clinical efficacy.

One of the key problems in treating laryngeal scar is that, by definition, scar tissue is dense and fibrotic. This makes it difficult for traditional topical medications to penetrate deeply into the affected tissue. The senior editor of this book (RTS) has utilized 5-FU as an injectable to prevent re-stenosis when treating posterior glottic stenosis with good results and no systemic side effects. A recent study by Gu *et al.*[25] investigated a new method for overcoming this problem. This involved the use of ethosomes; soft lipid vesicles containing a drug. They are able to penetrate tissues better than an aqueous solution, given their lipophilic nature. 5-FU was inserted into two different types of ethosomes that varied in diameter. All animals underwent surgical creation of laryngotracheal stenosis and were divided into four groups: (i) small ethosomes with drug, (ii) large ethosomes with drug, (iii) aqueous solution of drug, and (iv) saline control. The animals underwent a series of five percutaneous injections, each 5 days apart. All control animals died of airway obstruction prior to completing the study, with all treatment animals surviving. At the conclusion of the study, the Group A animals (small ethosomes) were found to have significantly less stenosis than either of the other two treatment groups, demonstrating that the smaller ethosomes provided greater treatment efficacy than injection of simple solution or even larger ethosomes.

Conclusions

Steroids, 5-FU, and MMC all show promise in alleviating scar of the larynx, and their potential efficacy may be increased when utilized with other modalities such as the laser. All three medications are commonly used today in practice, but no concrete clinical trials exist to provide standard guidelines on dosing and duration of therapy. Further investigation is needed to better define their place in the treatment of vocal fold scar.

References

1. Campagnolo AM, Tsuji DH, Sennes LU, Imamura R. Steroid injection in chronic inflammatory vocal fold disorders, literature review. *Rev Bras Otorrinolaringol* 2008; 74:926–932.

2. Wannmacher L, Ferreira MBC. Antiinflamatórios esteróides. In: Fuchs D, Wannmacher L, (Eds.). *Farmacologia Clínica* 2 edn. Rio de Janeiro: Guanabara Koogan 1998; pp. 194–202.

3. Campagnolo AM, Tsuji DH, Sennes LU, *et al.* Histologic study of acute vocal fold wound healing after corticosteroid injection in a rabbit model. *Ann Otol Rhinol Laryngol* 2010; 119:133–139.

4. Mortensen M, Woo P. Office steroid injections of the larynx. *Laryngoscope* 2006; 116:1735–1739.

5. Woo JH, Kim DY, Kim JW, *et al.* Efficacy of percutaneous vocal fold injections for benign laryngeal lesions: Prospective multicenter study. *Acta Otolaryngol* 2011; 131:1326–1332.

6. Filho PA, Rosen CA. Vocal fold plaque following triamcinolone. In: Sataloff RT, Hawkshaw MJ, Sataloff JB, *et al.* (Eds.) *Atlas of Laryngoscopy* 3 edn. San Diego, CA: Plural Publishing, Inc. 2013; pp. 289–290.

7. Li NYK, Chen F, Dikkers FG, Thibeault SL. Dose-dependent effect of mitomycin C on human vocal fold fibroblasts. *Head Neck* 2014; 36(3):401–410.

8. Hu D, Sires BS, Tong DC, *et al.* Effect of brief exposure to mitomycin C on cultured human nasal mucosa fibroblasts. *Ophthal Plast Reconstr Surg* 2000; 16:119–125.

9. Ferguson B, Gray SD, Thibeault S. Time and dose effects of mitomycin C on extracellular matrix fibroblasts and proteins. *Laryngoscope* 2005; 115:110–115.

10. Rahbar R, Jones DT, Nuss RC, *et al.* The role of mitomycin in the prevention and treatment of scar formation in the pediatric aerodigestive tract: friend or foe? *Arch Otolaryngol Head Neck Surg* 2002; 128:401–406.

11. Djordjevic B, Kim JH. Different lethal effects of mitomycin C and actinomycin D during the division cycle of HeLa cells. *J Cell Biol* 1968; 38:477–482.

12. Seong GJ, Park C, Kim CY, *et al.* Mitomycin-C induces the apoptosis of human Tenon's capsule fibroblast by activation of c-Jun N-terminal kinase 1 and caspase-3 protease. *Invest Ophthalmol Vis Sci* 2005; 46:3545–3552.

13. Talwar GP, Srivastava LM (Eds). *Textbook of Biochemistry and Human Biology.* New Delhi: Prentice–Hall of India Private Limited 2004.

14. Wu KY, Wang HZ, Hong SJ. Mechanism of mitomycin-induced apoptosis in cultured corneal endothelial cells. *Mol Vis* 2008; 14:1705–1712.

15. Hueman EM, Simpson CB. Airway complications from topical mitomycin C. *Otolaryngol Head Neck Surg* 2005; 133:831–835.

16. Roh JL, Kim DH, Rha KS, *et al.* Benefits and risks of mitomycin use in the traumatized tracheal mucosa. *Otolaryngol Head Neck Surg* 2007; 136:459–463.

17. Garrett CG, Soto J, Riddick J, *et al.* Effect of mitomycin-C on vocal fold healing in a canine model. *Ann Otol Rhinol Laryngol* 2001; 110(1):25–30.

18. Agrawal N, Morrison GA. Laryngeal cancer after topical mitomycin C application. *J Laryngol Otol* 2006; 120:1075–1076.

19. Pereira MC, Repka JCD, Camargo PAM, *et al*. Effect of topical mitomycin-C on total collagen deposits on the submucosa of intact vocal folds in swine. *Rev Col Bras* 2009; 36:236–240.

20. Fawaz SA, Sabri SM, Sweed AS, *et al*. Use of local mitomycin C in enhancing laryngeal healing after laser cordotomy: A prospective controlled study *Head Neck* 2013; Sept.:1248–1252.

21. Fitzpatrick RE. Treatment of Inflamed hypertrophic scars using intralesional 5-FU. *Dermatol Surg* 1999; 5:224–232.

22. Wurzer JC, Tallarida RJ, Sirover MA. New mechanism of action of the cancer chemotherapeutic agent 5-fluorouracil in human cells. *J Pharmacol Exp Ther* 1993; 269(1):39–43.

23. Fluorouracil. (2015). In: Epocrates Essentials. (Version 15.3) [Mobile application software]. Retrieved from http://www.epocrates.com/mobile/iphone [Accessed January 2016].

24. Baptistella E, Malagaia O, Czeczko NG, *et al*. Comparative study in swines' vocal cords healing after excision of fragment with CO_2 laser with mitomycin and 5-fluorouracil postoperative topical application. *Acta Cirurgica Brasileira* 2009; 24:14–18.

25. Gu J, Mao X, Li C, *et al*. A novel therapy for laryngotracheal stenosis: treatment with ethosomes containing 5-fluorouracil. *Ann Otol Rhinol Laryngol* 2015;1–6.

5

Vocal fold medialization

Farhad Chowdhury, Adam D. Rubin
and Robert T. Sataloff,

There can be multiple comorbid conditions associated with vocal fold scar that can affect a patient's symptoms and prognosis. Sulcus vocalis, a specific disorder related to vocal fold scar, can cause bowing of the medial edge of the vocal fold which causes glottic insufficiency described as a spindle-shaped glottis[1]. Vocal fold scar, and other associated abnormalities, can cause varying degrees of dysphonia such as breathiness, decreased volume, vocal fatigue, ineffective cough, and occasionally aspiration[2].

When addressing glottic insufficiency associated with vocal fold scar, several factors must be considered in selecting a type of medialization and the timing of the procedure. In many cases, surgery should not be performed until voice therapy has been tried. In some cases, strengthening vocal muscles and improving speaking technique results in improved voice quality and surgery is unnecessary – as discussed in a prior chapter. If surgery is needed, pre-operative voice therapy optimizes vocal use in the post-operative period. In some patients, improving glottic closure results in good voice and alleviates the need to operate to improve mucosal wave. In others, especially those with bilateral, opposing vocal fold scar, eliminating the glottic gap may make the voice worse and potentially strained in quality. Thyroid cartilage compression in the office is often helpful in surgical planning.

Surgical procedures that address the mucosal scar directly, such as an epithelial freeing technique and mucosal grafting (described in other chapters), should be considered prior to proceeding with medialization if it is clear that they will be required. In many cases improving the mucosal wave will also affect the glottic configuration and potentially the symptoms. Assessment of the glottic configuration is also important. In patients with paresis or paralysis in addition to scar, his/her voice may be normal during soft phonation but there may be insufficient lateral resistance to permit loud phonation. This problem is amenable to injection techniques or thyroplasty. If there is a gap in the middle of the musculomembranous vocal fold but good closure at the vocal process, implantation of a traditional thyroplasty prosthesis with a straight inner edge (such as a carved silastic block) is often less satisfactory than injection or use of a conformable prosthesis such as Gore-Tex® (Gore Medical, Flagstaff, AZ).

There are two common types of procedures to address glottic insufficiency: type-I thyroplasty (with or without arytenoid repositioning) and injection medialization. Type-I thyroplasty is typically considered a permanent procedure performed in the operating room via an external excision. Injection medialization can be performed in the office or operating room depending on the material used, surgeon preference, patient preference and patient tolerance. Various techniques are utilized for injection medialization (discussed below), but for all methods the material is injected lateral to the vocalis muscle at one or two locations (or more) depending on the response to injection and the degree of medialization needed. There are many injectable materials available, and there are pros and cons associated with each type and different durations of benefit, as described in detail below.

Injection laryngoplasty

Saline injection

Injectable saline can be utilized as a test injection lateral to the vocalis muscle prior to injecting a longer acting product. In the case of vocal fold scar, this may be particularly beneficial when it is unclear whether the vocal complaints will improve with correction of the glottic insufficiency. Saline is injected, typically in the office setting, using a trans-hyoid, trans-thyroid, or trans-cricothyroid membrane or transoral approach. Although the saline effects should last only hours, it is not unusual for patients to report residual improvement in glottic closure for several days or longer. The reasons are unknown.

Gelfoam injection

Gelfoam paste was introduced in 1978 by Schramm *et al.*[3]. This material is injected lateral to the vocalis musle, but it is temporary, resorbing in 2 to 8 weeks. It has been used for vocal fold injection for decades although it has never been approved formally by the FDA for this use. Gelfoam® (Pfizer, New York, NY) can be injected in the operating room or in the office. Office injection is performed per-orally, using a Brünings syringe with a curved needle, or transcutaneously like injection of Collagen (Dermalogen®, Collagenesis, Beverly, MA) and AlloDerm® (LifeCell Corporation, Branchburg, NJ) (discussed below). Although Gelfoam is considered temporary, it causes an inflammatory reaction that may lead to fibrosis. Scientific studies of laryngeal Gelfoam injection are wanting, and the assumption that laryngeal anatomy returns to normal following Gelfoam resorption remains unproven.

Carboxymethylcellulose

Carboxymethylcellulose is classified as a gel implant, and it is also used a carrier molecule coupled with calcium hydroxylapatite (CaHA). It is a commercially available injectable product approved for use in the vocal folds. It is a short-acting material that lasts 1–2 months[4] and can be injected using a 27-gauge needle using the standard techniques. Injection with this substance allows the patient to try out a voice with improved medialization and may be a precursor to a medialization thyroplasty. Unlike the other short-acting products, it is FDA-approved and inflammatory reactions have not been reported, so far.

Collagen

Ford and Bless have advocated the use of collagen for many conditions[5-9]. Collagen is in liquid form, which enhances the ease and accuracy of injection. Collagen may reduce scar formation because it stimulates production of collagenase. Bovine collagen was used initially but has been abandoned. Before injecting Bovine collagen, safety precautions such as skin testing are mandatory. However, human autologous and allogeneic collagen are available now and are superior to Bovine collagen for various reasons. Not only does the use of human material eliminate the severe reactions encountered occasionally with Bovine collagen, avoiding the need for skin testing, but human collagen may last longer, potentially making it more useful for lateral injection (medialization) than Bovine collagen[9-12].

A peroral technique as well as external techniques can be utilized. If the patient's gag reflex is too severe to permit peroral injection of collagen or other substances in an office setting, other techniques via the cricothyroid membrane or thyroid cartilage can be utilized. If these locations are too ossified to allow passage of a needle, it is often possible to inject the paraglottic space by passing a needle behind the posterior aspect of the thyroid lamina (Figure 5.1). Vocal fold injection also can be performed through the thyrohyoid membrane, using flexible nasolaryngoscopic visual guidance of course. Injection in the operating room using microdirect laryngoscopy with general anesthesia or local anesthesia with sedation is another option. Collagen injections appear to be efficacious in selected patients and are a valuable addition to the laryngologist's surgical armamentarium. Collagen, like Gelfoam paste, has not been FDA approved specifically for use in the larynx, although its use has become standard practice.

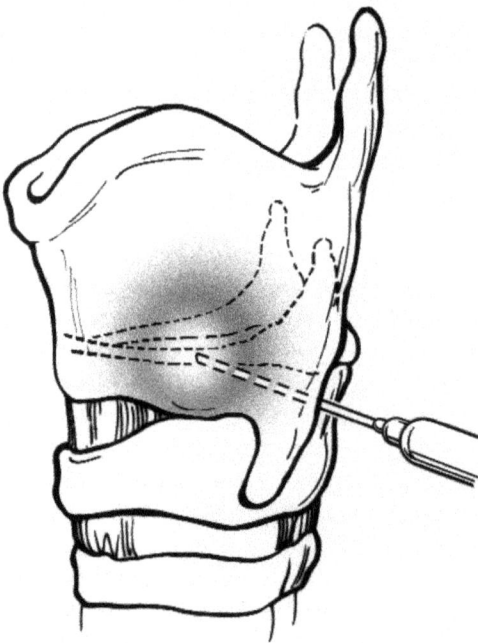

Figure 5.1 In most patients, the paraglottic space can be reached through a posterior approach, passing a needle behind the posterior border of the thyroid lamina and then angling it anteriorly and superiorly. Care should be taken to keep the needle close to the thyroid cartilage to help avoid injury to the piriform sinus or branches of the recurrent laryngeal nerve.

Cymetra micronized AlloDerm (LifeCell Corporation, Branchburg, NJ) is an acellular human tissue material that includes collagen, elastin, and proteoglycans. Its use in the larynx was reported by Passalaqua et al.[13]. They employed an external technique in which the thyroid lamina is pierced with a 22- or 24-gauge needle. Needle localization was confirmed using flexible nasolaryngoscopy, and

AlloDerm was injected laterally to treat conditions such as bowing (Figure 5.2). Like collagen, AlloDerm can be injected either through this external technique, through a peroral indirect technique in the office, or through direct laryngoscopy in the operating room.

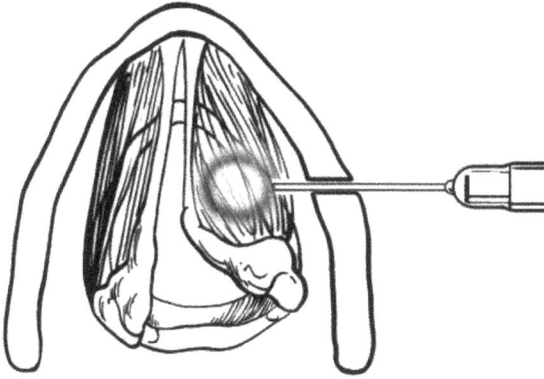

Figure 5.2 Injection of Alloderm, collagen, or other substances may be performed by passing a needle through the thyroid lamina. The point of insertion is usually about halfway between the anterior and posterior borders of the thyroid lamina and about 7–9 mm above the inferior border.

Fascia injection

Autologous fascia also has been advocated for vocal fold augmentation. Rihkanen advised cutting fascia into small pieces and delivering it through a Brünings syringe[14]. The principle problem with fascia is technical. If all of it is not cut into tiny pieces, it is very difficult to pass the fascia through the injection syringe. In our hands, during an early case, it obstructed the Brünings syringe so firmly that an attempt to pass it further forward resulted in breakage of the metal syringe. However, if the fascia is prepared properly, it can be a good material. Relatively little is resorbed, and excessive overcorrection should be avoided.

Hyaluronic acid

Hylauronic acid is a polysaccharide found in the extracellular matrix, and there are several commercial forms available including Restylane® (GalDerma, Lausanne, Switzerland) and Hylaform® (Genzyme, Washington, DC). It is FDA approved for use in cosmetic procedures, but it has been used in an off-label manor for injection medializations. There are reports of hypersensitivity and adverse reactions in its various uses[15]. A recent study on Restylane injection for vocal fold medialization found that the average duration of benefit was 12.2 weeks without adverse events[16]. It can be injected in the office or the operating room using the standard technique described previously.

Calcium hydroxyapatite

Calcium hydroxylapatite (CaHA), available in the form of Prolaryn Plus®, formerly known as Radiesse Voice®, (Merz, Raleigh, NC) is FDA approved for vocal fold augmentation. CaHA is a mineral component of bone that is biocompatible. The CaHA microspherules typically range in size from 25–45 microns and are suspended in an aqueous gel composed of water, glyceran, and sodium carboxymethylcellulose. Once injected, the body absorbs the gel carrier and the microspherules are left behind. The material is deliverable through a small-bore needle (25-gauge), and it is relatively durable. Carroll and Rosen recently showed its average length of benefit to be 18.6 months[17]. Injection laryngoplasty using calcium hydroxylapatite paste has been regarded as an effective and safe treatment for glottic insufficiency. However, in some patients CaHA can cause an intense inflammatory reaction (Figure 5.3a, Figure 5.3b), potentially migrate and compromise vocal fold function. While it has a place in the laryngologist's armamentarium, it should be used with full understanding of the potential serious adverse reactions, even though they do not occur often, and of the risk of at least minor impairment of vibratory function[18]. Clinicians should exercise caution when considering CaHA for vocal fold medialization.

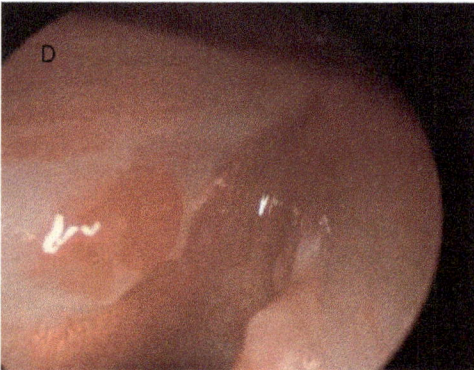

Figure 5.3a: A unilateral vocal fold granuloma is seen in the mid striking-zone in a patient who has undergone a unilateral injection laryngoplasty with calcium hydroxyapatite.

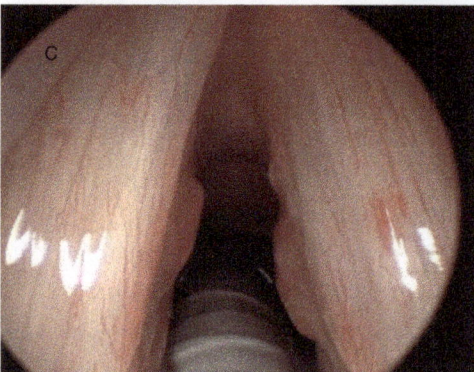

Figure 5.3b: Bilateral mid-striking zone granulomas are seen in a patient who has had a bilateral injection laryngoplasty with calcium hydroxyapatite.

Autologous fat

The first use of autologous fat in the larynx was reported by Dedo in 1975 for patients with laryngeal cancer[19]. He described the placement of a free fat graft under a mucosal advancement flap for creating a neo-vocal fold following vertical hemilaryngectomy. In many ways, the concept is analogous to the fat implantation described elsewhere in this book. Unfortunately, Dedo did not provide the number of patients, or any form of objective assessment; but he reported post-operative voices with minimal hoarseness or breathiness in all cases. This technique has not been used widely, and there are no recent reports of its continued use.

Human autologous fat injection into the larynx was first reported by Mikaelian, Lowry, and Sataloff in 1991[20] and subsequently by Brandenburg, Kirkham, and Koschkee[21]. These and subsequent reports dealt with autologous lipoinjection lateral to the vocalis muscle, which is different from lipoimplantation, described later. Fat requires overinjection by approximately 40%. The vocal fold should be convex at the conclusion of the procedure to account for expected resorption (Figure 5.4). This overinjection causes moderate, temporary dysphonia. If the voice is excellent at the end of the surgical procedure, a good final result is unlikely. In most cases, initial fat resorption occurs fairly quickly. Patients usually achieve a serviceable voice within 4 to 12 weeks. Additional changes occur over 6 to 12 months, occasionally necessitating reinjection in up to 1/3rd of patients[22].

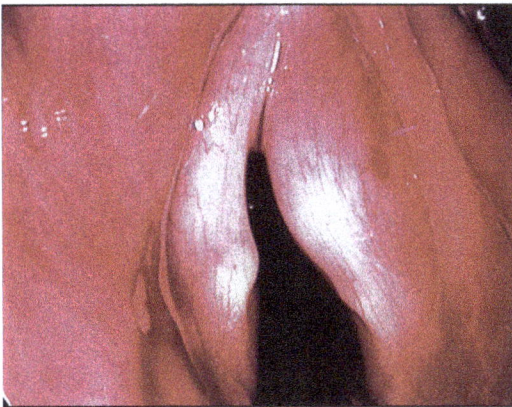

Figure 5.4: This 40-year-old marketing executive and avocational choir singer and musical theater performer had right recurrent nerve paralysis, apparently as a consequence of Lyme disease. Injection was performed near the middle of the right vocal fold *(arrow)*. This intra-operative photograph shows 30–40% overcorrection, the desired endpoint. The apparent bowing of the left vocal fold is an artifact.

Thyroplasty

Type I thyroplasty

Type I thyroplasty is an excellent approach to medialization. This procedure was popularized by Isshiki *et al.* in 1975[2,3] although the concept had been introduced early in the century by Payr[25]. Thyroplasty is performed under local anesthesia in nearly all cases. In classical thyroplasty, with the neck extended, a 4–5 cm incision is made horizontally at the midpoint between the thyroid notch and the lower rim of the thyroid cartilage. A rectangle of thyroid cartilage is cut on the involved side and removed. It begins approximately 5–7 mm lateral to the midline and is usually approximately 3–5 mm × 3–10 mm. The inferior border is located approximately 3 mm above the inferior margin of the thyroid cartilage. Care must be taken not to carry the rectangle too far posteriorly or it cannot be displaced medially. The cartilage is depressed inward, moving the vocal fold toward the midline. The wedge of silicone is then fashioned to hold the depressed cartilage in proper position (Figure 5.5). Since Isshiki's original description, most surgeons have preferred to remove the cartilage. Most preserve the inner perichondrium, although techniques that involve incisions through the inner perichondrium also have been used successfully.

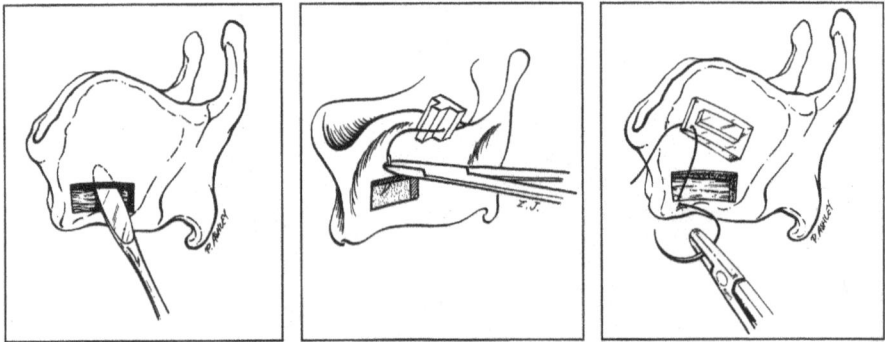

Figure 5.5: *(Left)* In Type I thyroplasty, cartilage is cut beginning 5–7 mm lateral to the midline. The window is about 3–5 mm × 3–10 mm. The window should be no more than 5 mm from the inferior border of the thyroid cartilage. After the cartilage cut has been completed, the inner perichondrium is elevated. This drawing illustrates correct window placement. *(Middle)* A silicone block is used to depress the cartilage into proper position, displacing the vocal fold medially. The silicone may be sutured to the cartilage. It is often necessary to taper the silicone anteriorly. This drawing also illustrates the most common errors in thyroplasty surgery, placing the window slightly too high and making the block too thick anteriorly. *(Right)* Appropriate thyroplasty window position and tapered prosthesis.

Surgeons also have used various other materials including autologous cartilage, hydroxylapatite, expanded polytetrafluoroethylene, and titanium[25-30]. Various additional technical modifications have been proposed as this technique has become more popular, and several varieties of pre-formed thyroplasty implant devices have been introduced commercially. Many of these modifications have proven helpful, especially techniques that obviate the need to carve individualized Silicone block implants, a technique that is often challenging for inexperienced thyroplasty surgeons. The use of Gore-Tex in the larynx was reported initially by Hoffman and McCulloch[29]. Since then, numerous reports have documented its efficacy[31,32]; material is easy to place, easy to adjust, and can be contoured to compensate for vocal fold bowing – which is of particular advantage when treating a scarred vocal fold. This procedure is performed under local anesthesia with sedation, and vocal fold position can be monitored by flexible laryngoscopy during phonatory response and at the end of the operation. Gore-Tex thyroplasty can be performed bilaterally at the same sitting and is particularly helpful in treating bilateral vocal fold bowing. In many cases, the procedure is performed as an outpatient, although overnight observation is appropriate if there is vocal fold swelling or any concern about airway compromise.

Arytenoid procedures

In some cases, more than one procedure is needed. In many cases, stages of surgery are planned from the outset. Many patients who need optimal voice (as compared to serviceable but dysphonic voices) require injection and thyroplasty or thyroplasty and arytenoid adduction/rotation or arytenoidopexy or medialization combined with reinnervation, or medialization combined with a procedure to restore mucosal wave. Arytneoid procedures and reinnervation procedures are reserved for vocal fold paralysis, and these procedures are discussed in more detail in other texts. One of the greatest challenges in scar management is the right procedure, or combination of procedures, and the order in which they should be used to achieve the best results possible.

References

1. Giovannie A, Chanterect C, Lagier A. Sulcus vocalis: a review. *Eur Arch Otolaryngol* 2007; 264(4):337–344.
2. Benniger MS, Alessi D, Archer S, *et al*. Vocal fold scarring: current concenpts and management. *Otolaryngol Head Neck Surg* 1996; 115(5):474–482.

3. Schramm VL, May MM, Lavorato AS. Gelfoam paste injection for vocal cord paralysis: temporary rehabilitation of glottic competence. *Laryngoscope* 1978; 88:1268–1272.

4. Kwon T, Buckmire R. Injection laryngoplasty for management of unilateral vocal fold paralysis. *Curr Opin Otolaryngol Head Neck Surg* 2004; 12(6):538–542.

5. Ford CN, Bless DM, Loftus JM. The role of injectable collagen in the treatment of glottic insufficiency: a study of 119 patients. *Ann Otol Rhinol Laryngol* 1992; 101(3):237–247.

6. Ford CN, Bless DM. Collagen injected in the scarred vocal fold. *J Voice* 1988; 1:116–118.

7. Ford CN, Bless DM. Selected problems treated by vocal fold injection of collagen. *Am J Otolaryngol* 1993; 14(4):257–261.

8. Cendron M, DeVore DP, Connolly R, *et al.* The biological behavior of autologous collagen injected into the rabbit bladder. *J Urol* 1995; 154:808–811.

9. Ford CN, Staskowski PA, Bless DM. Autologous collagen vocal fold injection: a preliminary clinical study. *Laryngoscope* 1995; 105(9):944–948.

10. DeVore DP, Hughes E, Scott JB. Effectiveness of injectable filler materials for smoothing wrinkle lines and depressed scars. *Med Prog Technol* 1994; 20:243–250.

11. Burstyn DG, Hagerman TC. Strategies for viral removal and inactivation. *Dev Biol Stand* 1996; 88:73–79.

12. DeVore DP, Kelman C, Fagien S, Casson P. Autologen: autologous, injectable dermal collagen. In: Bosniak S, (Ed.) *Ophthalmic Plastic and Reconstructive Surgery* Vol I. Philadelphia, PA: WB Saunders Company 1996: pp. 670–675.

13. Passalaqua P, Pearl A, Woo P, Ramospizarro CA. Direct transcutaneous translaryngeal injection laryngoplasty with AlloDerm. Presented at the 30th Annual Symposium: *Care of the Professional Voice*; June 16, 2001; Philadelphia, PA.

14. Rihkanen H. Vocal fold augmentation by injection of autologous fascia. *Laryngoscope* 1998; 108(1):51–54.

15. Shamanna SG, Bosch JD. Injection laryngoplasty: a serious reaction to hyaluronic acid. *J Otolaryngol Head Neck Surg* 2011; 40:E39–E42.

16. Halderman AA, Bryson PC, Benninger MS, Chota R. Safety and length of benefit of Restylan for office-based injection medialization – A retrospective review of one institution's experience. *J Voice* 2014; 28(5):631–635.

17. Carroll TL, Rosen CA. Long-term results of calcium hydroxylapatite for vocal fold augmentation. *Laryngoscope*. 2011; 121(2): 313–319.

18. Defatta RA, Chowdhury FR, Sataloff RT. Complications of injection laryngoplasty using calcium hydroxyapatite. *J Voice* 2012; 26(5):614–618

19. Kwon T, Buckmire R. Injection laryngoplasty for management of unilateral vocal fold paralysis. *Curr Opin Otolaryngol Head Neck Surg* 2004; 12(6):538–542.

20. Dedo H. A technique for vertical Hemilaryngectomy to prevent stenosis and aspiration. *Laryngoscope* 1975; 85:978–984.

21. Mikaelian D, Lowry LD, Sataloff RT. Lipoinjection for unilateral vocal cord paralysis. *Laryngoscope* 1991; 101:465–468.

22. Brandenburg J, Kirkham W, Koschkee D. Vocal cord augmentation with autologenous fat. *Laryngoscope* 1992; 102:495–500.
23. DeFatta RA, DeFatta RJ, Sataloff RT. Laryngeal lipotransfer: review of a 14-year experience. *J Voice* 2013; 27(4):512–515.
24. Isshiki N, Okamura H, Ishikawa T. Thyroplasty type I (lateral compression for dysphonia due to vocal cord paralysis or atrophy). *Acta Otolaryngol* 1975; 80:465–473.
25. Payr E. Plastik am schildknorpel zur Behebung der Folgen einseitiger Stimmband-lahmung. *Dtsch Med Wochensch* 1915; 43:1265–1270.
26. Cummings CW, Purcell LL, Flint PW. Hydroxylapatite laryngeal implants for medialization: preliminary report. *Ann Otol Rhinol Laryngol* 1993; 102:843–851.
27. Montgomery WW. Montgomery SK, Warren MA. Thyroplasty simplified. *Operative Tech Otolaryngol Head Neck Surg* 1993; 4:223–231.
28. Montgomery WW. Montgomery SK. Montgomery thyroplasty implant system. *Ann Otol Rhinol Laryngol* 1997; 106(suppl 107):1–16.
29. Flint PW, Corio RL, Cummings CW. Comparison of soft tissue response in rabbits following laryngeal implantation with hydroxylapatite, silicone rubber, and Teflon. *Ann Otol Rhinol Laryngol* 1997; 106:339–407.
30. McCulloch TM, Hoffman HT. Medialization laryngoplasty with expanded polytetrafluoroethylene-surgical technique and preliminary results. *Ann Otol Rhinol Laryngol* 1998; 107:427–432.
31. Friedrich G. Titanium vocal fold medializing implant: Introducing a novel implant system for external vocal fold medialization. *Ann Otol Rhinol Laryngol* 1998; 108:79–86.
32. Giovanni A, Vallicioni JM, Gras R, Zanaret M. Clinical experience with Gore-Tex for vocal fold medialization. *Laryngoscope* 1999; 109:284–288.
33. Zeitels SM, Mauri M, Dailey SH. Medialization laryngoplasty with Gore-Tex for voice restoration secondary to glottal incompetence: indications and observations. *Ann Otol Rhinol Laryngol* 2003; 112(2):180–184.

6

Epithelium freeing techniques

Aaron J. Jaworek, Mary J. Hawkshaw and
Robert T. Sataloff

Introduction

Despite advances in our understanding of the pathophysiology and histology of
vocal fold scar, the treatment of this condition remains one of the most problematic in phonomicrosurgery. The most important concept in understanding
vocal fold function and the dysfunction that accompanies vocal fold scar is
the body-cover theory[1]. The epithelial "cover" of the normal vocal fold vibrates
with minimal resistance from the transitional layers and "body" of the vocal
fold, which include the intermediate and deep layers of the lamina propria (the
vocal ligament) and the thyroarytenoid muscle because of pliability within the
superficial lamina propria (SLP). When the SLP is compromised, such as with
vocal fold scar and sulcus vocalis, the epithelium can no longer glide freely over
the deeper layers of the vocal fold. This impairs mucosal wave propagation producing the dysphonia and glottic insufficiency that often are associated with
scar. Surgery limited strictly to the epithelium and the SLP, a relatively hypo-
cellular zone deficient in collagen[2,3] is less likely to cause symptomatic scar than
surgery involving the deeper layers. For this reason, accessing pathology through
this layer with minimal collateral damage has been the primary focus in the
development of surgical techniques to prevent scar, and restoration of pliability
to this region has been a primary goal in the development of surgery to treat
scar. However, it is important to remember that restoration of mucosal wave is

only one component of scar management. Correction of glottic insufficiency, or partial correction in patients with bilateral opposing scar, also is essential and may involve less risk than some procedures to restore mucosal wave. Management of glottic insufficiency in patients with scar is discussed elsewhere in this book. The decision whether to correct glottic insufficiency or mucosal wave first, or whether to correct them simultaneously, must be individualized. If good voice is achieved through thyroid cartilage compression in the office, medialization without risking mucosal wave surgery may be sufficient. If thyroid cartilage compression produces strained voice because of bilateral vocal fold scar, more complex, staged procedures may be needed to achieve optimal voice.

Trans-oral

Subepithelial infusion

Elevation of the vocal fold epithelium via the SLP can be accomplished in some patients using subepithelial infusion. This technique involves needle tip insertion into the region of the superficial lamina propria followed by injection of a biologically inert substance, such as normal saline with or without epinephrine, a glucocorticoid (e.g. dexamethasone), or other material (Figure 6.1). The resultant hydrodissection serves as a diagnostic tool and therapeutic vehicle. It can help to delineate the extent of scar, lyse minor adhesions, and identify any areas that might be densely adherent to the vocal ligament. In some cases, infusion into the SLP is sufficient to release a scar band or adhesion without the need for further surgical intervention.

Zeitels *et al.* described this technique using normal saline as a means to elevate a variety of lesions prior to their excision[4,5]. They were able to penetrate different layers of the lamina propria from just below the basement membrane of the epithelium to the deep lamina propria. They reported that some scar and sulci required an increased depth of penetration of the needle in order to elevate the lesion successfully with this approach. By expanding this space, the surgeon can delineate the boundaries differentiating normal and abnormal pliability to minimize the surface area of the epithelium to be excised and to locate adhesions to be lysed. In this manner, infusion has been useful to identify pathology that was not seen readily on prior evaluations of the vocal folds both in the office and in the operating room. The senior author (RTS) also has found that in some cases, small adhesions that do not elevate easily with hydrodissection can be

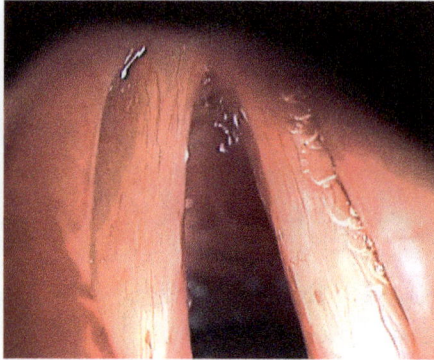

A

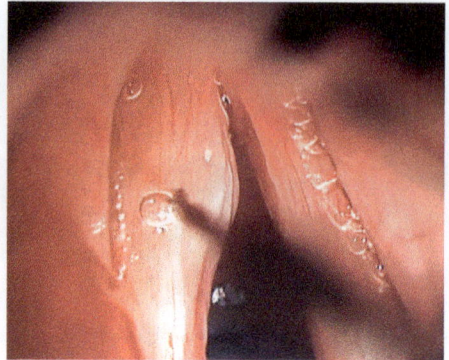

B

Figure 6.1 (**a**) An area of scar is visualized along the left vocal fold with direct laryngoscopy. (**b**) Subepithelial injection with dexamethasone is used to elevate the scar. (**c**) Multiple injections may be required to adequately disperse the dexamethasone, hydrodissect under the epithelium, and lyse adhesions.

(Reproduced with permission from: Sataloff RT, Chowdhury F, Joglekar S, and Hawkshaw MJ. Chapter 21: Vocal Fold Scar. In Sataloff, R.T. *Atlas of Endoscopic Laryngeal Surgery*. Jaypee Brothers Medical Publishers Ltd. 2011, pp. 123–125.)

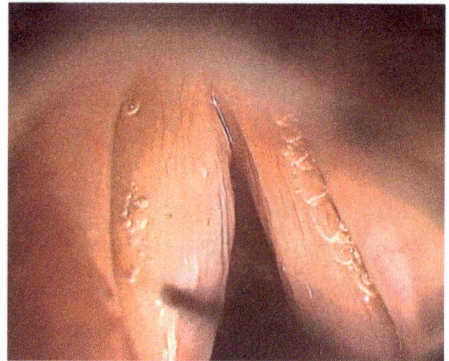

C

lysed with the sharp edge of the infusion needle, obviating the need for a larger incision or more extensive surgery.

Infusion of saline into the SLP also has been used as a "heat sink" during laser treatment of the vocal fold[5]. This can be accomplished directly when using the carbon dioxide (CO_2) laser, since its chromophore is water. The subepithelial saline also can serve as a nontargeted heat sink when using photoangiolytic lasers, such as the potassium titanyl phosphate (KTP) and pulsed dye lasers (PDL), because their chromophore is oxyhemoglobin. Additionally, the infusion can place areas of scar under tension, allowing for more precision when using the laser and reducing thermal injury to healthy adjacent tissue. Infusion can facilitate excision of scar when using cold instruments, as well.

One pitfall with subepithelial infusion is that overinjection can create a false impression that a lesion is larger or penetrates more deeply than it does, or it can obscure the lesion. It is important to maintain balance between utility and distortion with this procedure. If the vocal fold is overinjected, aqueous solutions such as saline and dexamethasone often can be aspirated or expressed with gentle instrumentation through the needle injection site.

The principle of expanding SLP volume and decreasing inflammation also has been employed in an effort to reduce the formation of scar postoperatively, although definitive evidence supporting the efficacy of this common practice is wanting. Wang *et al.* reviewed the literature available on this important topic[6]. By injecting a glucocorticoid such as dexamethasone, inhibition of fibroblast proliferation might be achieved resulting in a reduction of overabundant collagen synthesis, the primary constituent of scar[7]. Similarly, collagen, hyaluronic acid, fat, and fascia, among other substances, have been injected or implanted into the SLP to act as volume expanders, theoretically softening and releasing existing scar, and reducing subsequent scar formation by a variety of mechanisms[8-13]. When considering infusion of a substance into the SLP, the surgeon should be aware of the material's potential for positive and negative consequences with respect to ease of injection, reabsorption potential, inflammatory response, and goals of surgery[14]. A well-documented example of how a lack of sufficient understanding of the unfavorable consequences of an injectable substance can influence outcomes, is the formation of granulomas with Teflon[15,16]. Calcium hydroxylapatite occasionally causes similar problems when used for injection laryngoplasty[17,18]. It is helpful to understand the biocompatibility, viscoelastic properties, and duration of effect for the variety of materials used in vocal fold augmentation (Tables 6.1, 6.2, Figure 6.2).

Table 6.1 Biocompatibility of materials used for vocal fold augmentation.

Biocompatible	Variable Biocompatibility
Normal saline	Hyaluronic acid (e.g. Restylane, Juvederm)
Autologous fat	Gelatine (e.g. Gelfoam)
Autologous fascia	Collagen (e.g. Cymetra)
	Carboxymethylcellulose (e.g Prolaryn Gel®)
	Calcium hydroxylapatite (e.g. Prolaryn Plus®)

Table 6.2 Duration of common materials used for vocal fold injection augmentation.

Material	Duration of Effect
Normal saline	1–3 hours
Gelatin (e.g. Gelfoam)	1–3 months
Carboxymethylcellulose (e.g. Prolaryn Gel®)	1–3 months
Hyaluronic acid (e.g. Restylane, Juvederm)	3–6 months
Collagen (e.g. Cymetra)	6–12 months
Calcium hydroxylapatite (e.g. Prolaryn Plus®)	12–24 months
Autologous fat	Permanent (30–50% resorption)
Autologous fascia	Permanent

Source: King JM and Simpson CB. Modern injection augmentation for glottic insufficiency. *Curr Opin Otolaryngol Head Neck Surg* 2007; 15:153–158

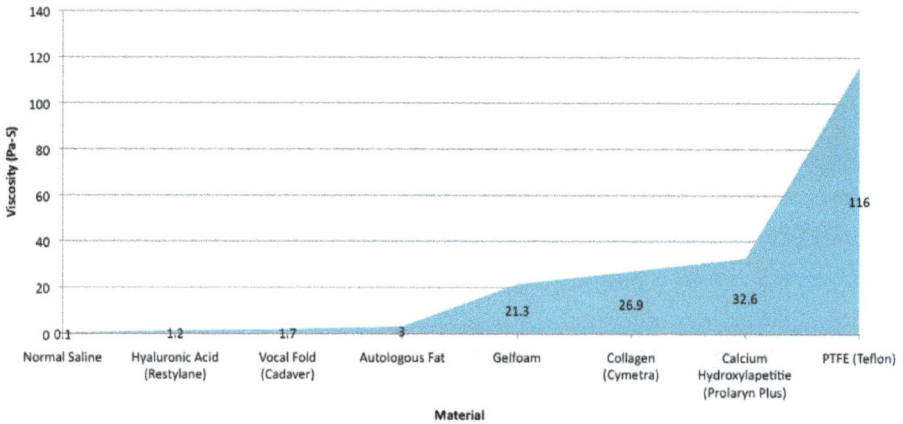

Figure 6.2 Graph showing the viscosity (Pa-s) of materials used for vocal fold augmentation relative to the native vocal fold (cadaver) at 10 Hz. Teflon has been included for comparison only. Note that hyaluronan derived substances and autologous fat most closely resemble the native vocal fold viscoelastic properties.

1. Lisi C, Hawkshaw MJ, and Sataloff RT. Viscosity of materials for laryngeal injection: A review of current knowledge and clinical implications. *J Voice* 2013; 27(1): 119–123.

2. Chan RW and Titze I. Viscosities of implantable biomaterials in vocal fold augmentation surgery. *Laryngoscope* 1998; 108: 725: 731.

Studies have shown hyaluronan-derived substances to resemble most closely the vibratory characteristics of the native vocal fold[12,14,19]. Of the available products on the market, *Juvéderm®* (Allergan, Irvine) was found to have the closest viscoelastic properties. Although well tolerated in the majority of cases, there is still a potential risk of an inflammatory response with hyaluronic acid. Also, its effect is temporary. As an alternative, the senior author (RTS) has had success using autologous fat harvested from the abdomen for vocal fold injection laryngoplasty and for implantation at the medial edge[17,19,20]. With fat, there is no risk of a foreign body reaction and, like hyaluronic acid, it has viscoelastic properties closely resembling the native vocal fold[14]. Most importantly, after accounting for some absorption, the effect is expected to be permanent.

Selection of material and the amount to be injected are dependent on the severity of any glottic gap that has resulted from vocal fold scar, atrophy, or paresis. In patients in whom a large glottic gap is present, focusing efforts solely on epithelial freeing will not be sufficient to close the gap. A vocal fold injection usually should not be performed simultaneously with mucosal freeing unless a small volume of material is injected laterally. The medial displacement of the vibratory margin caused by injection medialization (such as with routine over-injection of fat) counteracts scar elevation of the medial edge of the vocal fold. In general, procedures to restore the mucosal wave and medialize the vocal fold should be staged. One procedure that has treated vocal fold scar successfully in the presence of glottic insufficiency in the senior author's (RTS) experience is autologous fat implantation[20,22,24,25], which will be discussed in greater detail later in this chapter.

When determining the best surgical approach to a vocal fold with substantial scar and a glottic gap, it is important to understand the contributions of each to the dysphonia. While medialization can improve volume and reduce vocal fatigue and breathiness in the presence of scar, it can intensify the harsh strained phonation contributed by the scarred vocal fold(s). This observation illustrates the importance of adequate preoperative evaluation with strobovideolaryngoscopy and with manual compression of the thyroid cartilage. A novice mistake is to proceed with complete medialization while failing to address bilateral scar along the medial edge, only to encounter a disappointing postoperative result with increased phonation threshold pressures and phonatory effort, despite an apparently "good result" on stroboscopy with complete glottic closure.

Microflap and mini-microflap

A second method of elevating vocal fold epithelium endoscopically involves making an incision through the vocal fold epithelium. Although the microflap (Figure 6.3) technique that was first introduced in the early 1980s has been replaced by the mini-microflap (Figure 6.4) since the early 1990s for treating the majority of benign vocal fold masses, microflap may prove beneficial in lifting dense or adherent scar in some cases[20,21]. Because the classic microflap requires that the overlying epithelium be preserved and that the incision and dissection extend beyond the area of pathology, it is often not well suited for addressing scar in the absence of other pathology. What led to the senior author's development of the mini-microflap procedure was the observation that the standard microflap sometimes resulted in stiffness or the formation of scar not only in the original area of pathology, but also beyond its boundaries.

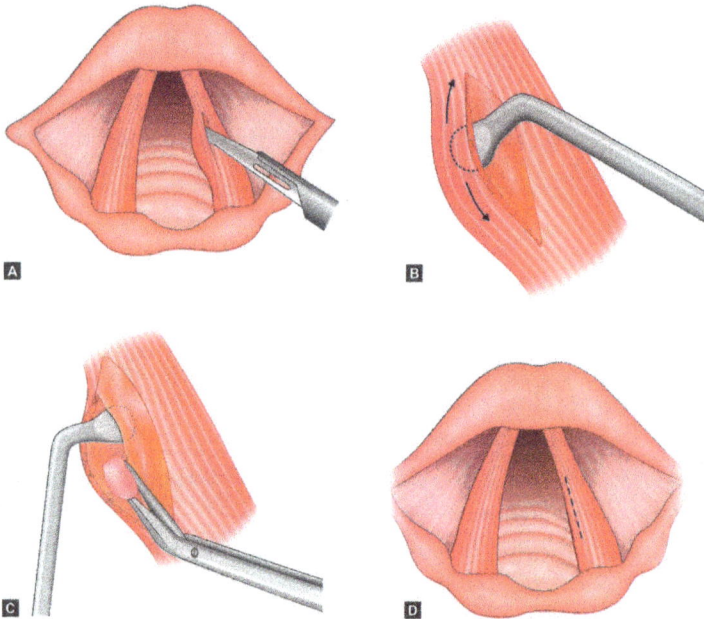

Figure 6.3 Microflap procedure. In this technique, a superficial incision is made in the superior surface of the true vocal fold (**a**). Blunt dissection is used to elevate the mucosa from the lesion (**b**), minimizing trauma to the fibroblast-containing layers of the lamina propria. Only pathologic tissue is excised under direct vision (**c**). Mucosa is reapproximated (**d**) without violating the leading edge. This technique is no longer recommended by this author.
(Reproduced with permission from: Sataloff R. T., *Surgical Techniques in Otolaryngology-Head and Neck Surgery: Laryngeal Surgery*. Philadelphia, Delhi, London. Jaypee Brothers Medical Publishers. 2014)

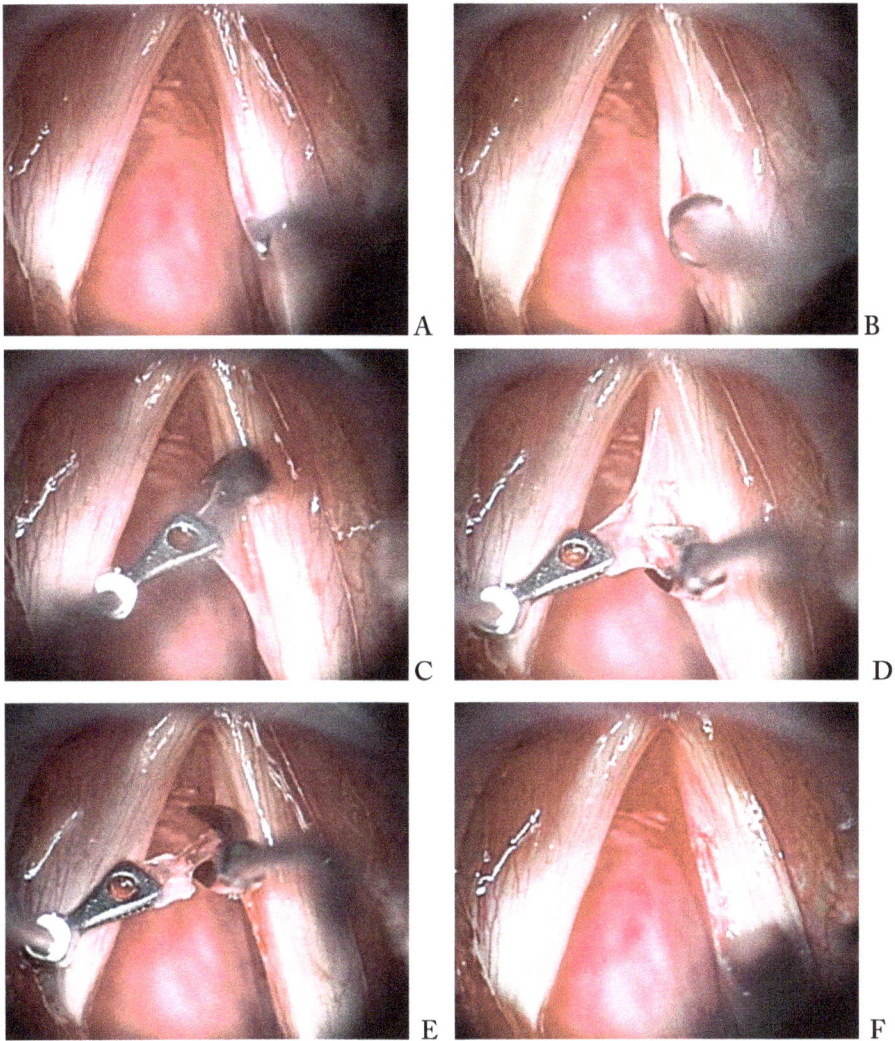

Figure 6.4 (a) In elevating a mini-microflap, an incision is made with a straight knife at the junction of the mass/scar and normal tissue. Small vertical anterior and posterior incisions may be added at the margins of the mass if necessary, usually using straight scissors. **(b)** The mass is separated by blunt dissection, splitting the superficial layer of the lamina propria and preserving it as much as possible. This dissection can be performed with a spatula, blunt ball dissector, or scissors (as illustrated). **(c–e)**

The lesion is stabilized and a pair of scissors (straight or curved) is used to excise the lesion, preserving as much adjacent mucosa as possible. Some lesions act as a tissue expander, and it is possible to create an inferiorly based mini-microflap. **(f)** The mini-microflap is replaced over the surgical defect, establishing primary closure and acting as a biological dressing.

(Reproduced with permission from: Sataloff RT, Chowdhury F, Joglekar S, and Hawkshaw MJ. Chapter 13: Vocal Fold Cysts. In Sataloff, R.T. *Atlas of Endoscopic Laryngeal Surgery*. Jaypee Brothers Medical Publishers Ltd. 2011, pp. 66–67.)

A microflap involves a small incision ideally along the superior surface of the vocal fold at the junction of normal and abnormal tissue. The direction of the incision is oriented parallel to the medial edge of the vocal fold. The senior author (RTS) accomplishes this task using a straight microlaryngeal blade, but it can be executed with the laryngeal sickle knife, as well. When using the straight microlaryngeal blade, the direction of the incision is from anterior to posterior using a gentle "sawing" motion, rather than pulling the knife posteriorly – which can result in an uncontrolled extension of the planned incision. Care must be taken to place the tip of the blade no deeper than the SLP to avoid trauma to the deeper layers of the lamina propria. When using the laryngeal sickle knife, a path of incision from posterior to anterior may provide optimal visualization. A slight sawing motion also is used, along with gentle force directed cranially towards the surgeon in order to tent the epithelium away from the deeper layers of the vocal fold as the incision is being made. The tip of the blade should be visible through the epithelial layer to ensure proper depth of the instrument. The incision should be made just large enough to allow for elevation of the desired flap, lysis of scar adhesions, and/or infusion of a material targeted at minimizing the risk of subsequent scar formation. Maintaining the position of an infused or implanted material is difficult with this approach, a problem that led to the development of the fat implantation technique described later in this chapter.

Prior to making the incision, subepithelial infusion into the SLP can be completed for the indications discussed earlier. A subepithelial infusion with a vasoconstricting agent, such as normal saline with 1:10,000 epinephrine, can be used for hypervascular vocal folds or when other concerns about excessive bleeding exist. Normal saline alone may have a similar effect short term through direct compression of the microvasculature in the vocal fold.

Following the incision, access to the SLP is achieved with insertion of a phonomicrosurgical instrument into the incision and gentle undermining within the SLP until a small pocket has been created. Instruments that have been used for this purpose include microscissors, a right angle microdissector, the round-tipped ball probe, a spatula, and a Sataloff flap knife (Integra, Plainsboro), among others. The smallest amount of dissection should be completed to accomplish the desired task. Experience with this technique is invaluable to minimize trauma to the overlying epithelium, as well as to the intermediate and deep layers of the lamina propria. Except in cases of thick scar, visualizing the dissecting instrument under the flap indicates that it is placed properly within the SLP. Particularly when approaching the medial edge of the vocal fold or when the epithelium becomes less pliable due to dense scar, the instrument should be pressed gently against the deeper layers of the vocal fold (which already are involved with scar). Tenting the epithelium is more likely to tear the flap.

The mini-microflap requires far less dissection in the SLP than a microflap. Mini-microflap also allows for the excision of scar and abnormal epithelium so involved with scar that it is not pliable even when mobilized from the deeper layers of the lamina propria. The mini-microflap can be used to lyse adhesions and excise scar bands, also. The disadvantage of the microflap and mini-microflap for scar is that they often do not allow for the subsequent infusion or implantation of a substance into the SLP near the surgical site because of extrusion.

The development of the transoral endoscopic fat implantation technique addressed the issue of preserving epithelium while lysing severe scar, and retaining implanted material, so long as there is reasonable epithelial pliability. When there is not, epithelial replacement such as with a buccal graft should be considered, as discussed elsewhere in this book.

Fat implantation

Autologous fat implantation along the medial edge of the vocal fold was first described in 1995 by the senior author (RTS) to achieve elevation and volume expansion of the SLP, improve glottic insufficiency, and recover some of the vibratory characteristics lost by a vocal fold affected by scar[21].

Successful execution of the fat implantation technique requires special attention to a few key steps (Figure 6.5):

1) A small incision is made through the epithelium laterally along the superior surface of the vocal fold.

2) An access tunnel is created toward the medial edge of the vocal fold with a blunt-tipped dissector. Instruments are passed through the access tunnel to create a pocket on the medial surface of the vocal fold.

3) The medial pocket should extend to the superior aspect of the vibratory margin and inferiorly for at least 3–5 mm to encompass the entire medial surface ordinarily involved in creating the mucosal wave vertical phase difference during phonation. Dissection along the superior surface of the vocal fold, except at the 2–3 mm access tunnel, should be avoided to prevent extrusion or migration of fat from the medial edge into this region.

4) In the senior author's (RTS) experience, abdominal fat harvested via the largest liposuction cannula (8–10 mm) has proved to be more effective than en bloc resection of fat in order to distribute the fat evenly within the SLP and to avoid a lumpy vocal fold medial edge.

5) A Brünings syringe is effective for delivering the harvested fat to the pocket along the medial edge of the vocal fold. The path of the needle during implantation should be at an angle rather than perpendicular to the vocal fold in order to minimize extrusion of the fat. The access tunnel with this angled approach produces a "trap door" effect to help seal in the implanted fat. The more the medial pocket is filled, the more firmly the self-closing "trap door" is sealed by medial distention of the mucosa. Occasionally, the senior author (RTS) has created a slight bend in the injector needle if the correct angle for fat delivery cannot be achieved with a straight needle.

6) Other authors have noted that with microflaps, if the flap becomes unstable or freely mobile, fibrin glue or a small micro-suture can be used to secure the flap[23]. However, this is not routinely needed or recommended by the senior author (RTS) when using the autologous fat implantation technique. Moreover, fibrin glue is usually not effective, and tying a suture creates small holes at the suture site through which fat may extrude.

It is important to appreciate that with this technique, return of the mucosal wave usually does not begin until 3–6 months following the procedure, and the optimum voice outcome may not be achieved until 6–12 months or more[24]. Reporting on the first eight patients who underwent fat implantation with a mean follow-up of 23 months, Neuenschwander et al. observed statistically significant improvement in glottic closure, mucosal wave, and stiffness[25]. There was statistically significant improvement in all five parameters of the Grade, Roughness, Breathiness, Asthenia, and Strain (GRBAS) rating scale, as well. The only complication in this series was an abdominal hematoma requiring evacuation.

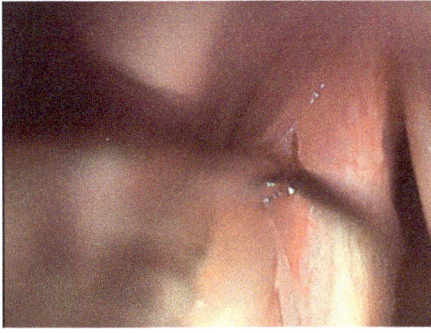

A

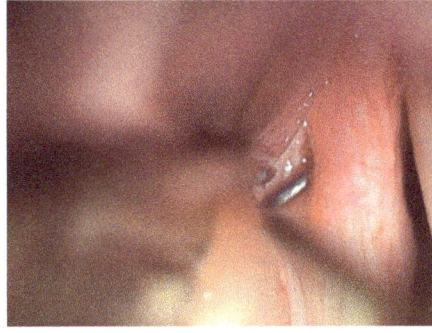

B

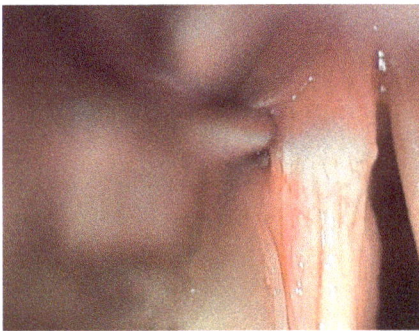

C

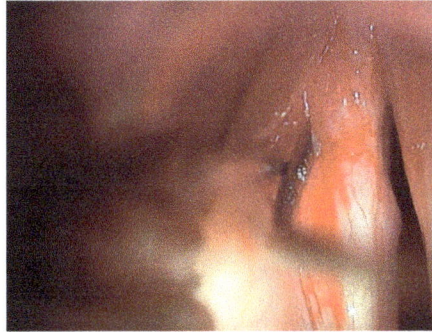

D

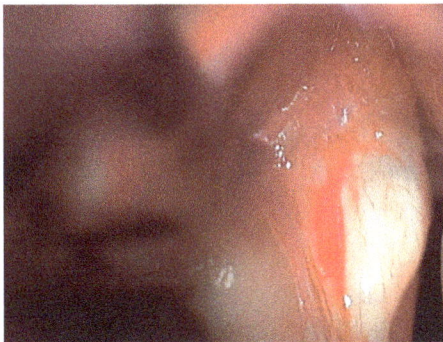

E

Figure 6.5 (a) A small incision is made on the superior surface of the scarred vocal fold. (b) A narrow access tunnel is excavated to provide access to the medial edge. (c) Through the access tunnel, an angled instrument is used to elevate a pocket. It is essential that the mucosa along the medial and inferior margins be kept intact. (d) A Brünings syringe with the largest needle is passed through the tunnel and used to deposit fat in the pocket. (e) When the needle is removed, the small access tunnel closes spontaneously, preventing extrusion of the fat. Fat should not extrude even when pressure is placed against the medial margin. If fat extrusion occurs, a suture can be placed.

Mucosal slicing technique

A very different approach to releasing epithelium for vocal fold sulci has been described by Pontes and Behlau and is called the "sulcus mucosal slicing technique"[26]. Through the creation of three or four mucosal cuts of varying sizes along the medial edge of the vocal fold, they have demonstrated improvement in vibratory function in selected patients[27]. The goal of the surgery is to interrupt the longitudinal tension produced by the presence of the sulcus, as well as to promote mucosal vibration by bringing the pliable ventricular tissue to participate in the sound source. They reported that this technique can also reduce a glottic gap. Complications were rare but included granuloma and synechiae, the latter being described as soft and easily lysed without recurrence[26].

The basic steps of the mucosal slicing technique include the following:

1) A parallel incision is made ~1 mm above the superior lip of the sulcus (cranial orientation), extending from 1 mm from the anterior commissure to 1 mm from the vocal process of the arytenoid cartilage.

2) Mucosa is detached up to 2 mm below the inferior lip of the sulcus, without touching the vocal ligament. Thick tissue flaps are advocated to preserve vascular properties and avoid necrosis.

3) Four to five vertical incisions of different lengths are made in the detached mucosa along the length of the sulcus, producing three to four segments of mucosa of different sizes.

4) The mucosal segments are positioned without suturing.

5) The authors advocate completing the procedure bilaterally in one stage regardless of sulcus asymmetry.

6) Three days of voice rest, 14 days of prednisone, and intensive voice therapy beginning on day 4 are recommended postoperatively.

Evaluation of acoustical parameters revealed that the mucosal slicing procedure offered overall vocal quality improvement 6 months after intervention with intensive voice therapy in 9 of 10 treated patients[26]. Moreover, stroboscopic examination of the vocal folds 1 year after surgery revealed better vibratory patterns and improved glottic closure in the same nine patients.

Trans-cervical

Laryngofissure

Laryngofissure procedure has been described extensively since its introduction in 1788 by Pellatone for multiple applications including the treatment of severe vocal fold scar. It allows for direct visualization of the vocal folds via an open surgical approach and access to the SLP via the anterior commissure. The obvious disadvantage is that it is more invasive than endoscopic surgery, possibly resulting in a longer recovery period, and sometimes it requires that a tracheotomy be placed, albeit temporarily. The senior author (RTS) has performed laryngofissures without tracheotomy and sometimes under local anesthesia with sedation. Laryngofissures often are reserved for patients for whom less invasive surgical approaches (i.e. endoscopic) have failed. Details of the procedure are discussed elsewhere in this book. Once adequate exposure has been obtained, a pocket at least 3–5 mm in height can be developed, ideally between the epithelium and the vocal ligament. In many cases, due to the extent of scar – such as with laryngeal trauma – the pocket is created either between the vocal ligament and the thyroarytenoid muscle, or deep to the residual thyroarytenoid muscle. A durable tunnel must be elevated that will support implantation of fat or a pedicled flap from one of the strap muscles, if desired[28].

Gray's minithyrotomy

A less invasive direct access approach to the SLP, coined "Gray's minithyrotomy," (GMT) was introduced in 1999, permitting surgical manipulation of the vocal fold lamina propria in a subepithelial plane through a window in the thyroid cartilage[29]. It has been adopted by many laryngologists who have reported their experiences with this technique[30,31].

Reported benefits of this approach include access for microscopic instruments with the surgeon's hands close to the tissue of interest, avoidance of intralaryngeal mucosal incisions, and lining up the direction of dissection in an anterior-to-posterior orientation[29]. Once access has been obtained, any material can be injected or implanted based on the same principles as described earlier. Like the laryngofissure, GMT also affords the ability to insert a perichondrium flap or a pedicled muscle flap when extra tissue volume is needed, such as with cases of severe scarring of the vocal fold. Thyroid ala perichondrium (TAP) flaps and composite thyroid ala perichondrium (CTAP) flaps have been investigated in vivo in canine models by Dailey *et al.*[32,33]. Paniello *et al.* opined that the minithyrotomy procedure is ideal for "lateralizing scar" in the paraglottic space, since it can be addressed through the same incision[31]. Harvesting fat for implantation during GMT also does not require a second surgical site. Other potential benefits that have been cited depend greatly on surgical technique and experience with this and related procedures. It has been described as being less ideal for treating scar caused by "stripping" and re-epithelialization because the subepithelial layer often is too thin imparting a higher risk of perforation.

The basic steps of the Gray's minithyrotomy include the following:

1) A 1–2 cm horizontal incision is made in the anterior neck overlying the thyroid cartilage.

2) Fat from the subcutaneous layer of the anterior neck is harvested for implantation, if desired.

3) After exposing the thyroid cartilage, the minithyrotomy is created by cutting or drilling a 3–4 mm window of thyroid cartilage slightly off the midline of the anterior commissure area.

   • Paniello *et al.* proposed that the hole be aligned with the vocal fold, rather than perpendicular to the thyroid cartilage surface. The center of the hole should be 3–4 mm lateral to midline and 3–4 mm superior to the inferior edge of the thyroid cartilage[31].

   • The location of the minithyrotomy also can be determined by passing a 22 gauge needle through the cartilage at the planned site of entry. Ideally, the needle should enter the vocal fold in the SLP just deep to the leading edge, or slightly lower.

   • The correct position can be confirmed with laryngoscopy by a variety of methods including either transnasal or transoral flexible laryngoscopy, or using a transoral direct suspension laryngoscopy approach with a telescope or microscope.

4) A pocket is developed parallel to the vector of the vocal fold, taking care to avoid creating a pocket that is too large anteriorly. When this occurs, too much of the implanted material will accumulate anteriorly, which may result in a strained voice.

5) After the tunnel has been created, a straight ear pick is used to extend the subepithelial tunnel from the anterior commissure to the vocal process.

6) Starting with the needle each time, this sequence is repeated until the needle can be passed easily through the entire length of the musculomembranous vocal fold within the infraglottic and leading edge areas.

- For scar or sulcus, sharp dissection is preferable to blunt dissection. This can be facilitated by using a duckbill, a Sheehy ("Gimmick") elevator, or small, curved Bellucci scissors[30,31].

- Ultimately, the final pocket should include the area of scar, the free edge, and 2–3 mm inferior to the scar.

- Dissection along the superior aspect of the vocal fold should be avoided when possible.

7) The desired material is implanted within the pocket, usually fat, fascia, or both.

8) Fibrin glue or bone wax may be used to help seal the minithyrotomy site.

9) The neck is closed in layers with or without the placement of a small drain. A drain is preferable to reduce the risk of subcutaneous emphysema when penetration through the vocal fold epithelium occurs.

When the procedure was first introduced, Gray acknowledged that connecting the tunnels proved to be the most challenging step due to the lack of ideal instruments small enough to fit through the minithyrotomy and subepithelial pocket[29]. A small alligator strut was found to be useful by Paniello et al. during this step. Dailey et al. have developed a set of instruments to improve the success of this procedure[33].

Gray et al. originally described this procedure in conjunction with fat implantation; however, other materials such as fascia or injectables can be considered. Paniello et al. described insertion of harvested fat after cutting it into 1–2 cm × 3 mm strips[31]. To account for resorption, overcorrection is needed (typically 40–50%). Mallur et al. used a 19 gauge angiocatheter for fat implantation in their case series[30]. Additionally, fat implantation using a Brünings syringe can be accomplished in a similar manner to the transoral approach described by Sataloff et al.

In small case series, outcomes following GMT have been promising. Paniello et al. noted voice improvement in the third month following the procedure that was sustained at 6 months using VHI, CAPE-V, and self-rated voice severity scores[31]. In those patients with scar as the primary indication for surgery, all but 2 had improved mucosal waves at follow up. The reported complications included fat extrusion 2/21 (9.5%) and mucosal perforation 3/21 (14%). If a small perforation is made, outer perichondrium from the thyroid cartilage can be used as an inlay graft through the minithyrotomy tunnel to cover the defect. In general, the larger the perforation, the greater the risk of implant extrusion.

Mallur *et al.* analyzed 13 GMT procedures using VHI-10, self-reported voice outcomes, mucosal wave, and glottic closure[30]: 6 of the 13 (46%) cases had improved VHI-10 scores, (3 were unchanged, 4 were worse); 7 (54%) cases had improved self-reported outcomes. Mucosal wave improved in 7 of 17 (41%) vocal folds (3 vocal folds could not be visualized). Glottic closure improved in 7 of 13 cases (54%). Complications in this series occurred in 5 of 16 (31%) cases. They were neck ecchymosis, subcutaneous emphysema with seroma and abscess, tongue paresthesia and taste alteration, wound dehiscence, and aspiration pneumonia.

Microendoscopy of Reinke's space (MERS)

The microendoscopy of Reinke's space (MERS) technique represents a modification of the Gray's minithyrotomy procedure by providing direct visualization into the surgically created minithyrotomy with a microendoscope or sialendoscope[34,35]. At the present time, it is in early stages of development, and future studies are needed to establish its efficacy among the available options for treating vocal fold scar, a condition in which Reinke's space often is absent.

The basic steps of microendoscopy of Reinke's space include the following:

1) Initial dissection is carried out similar to a thyroplasty or GMT to expose the thyroid cartilage and cricothyroid membrane. Modifications for a minimally invasive approach are likely to be investigated.

2) MERS access points include:

- **Access point #1**: A 5 mm fenestration (thyrotomy) located 6 mm lateral to the midline and 6 mm above the lower border of the thyroid cartilage.

- **Access point #2**: A small puncture in the cricothyroid membrane.

3) A 27-gauge needle followed by a stylet is inserted through access point #1, and concurrent imaging from the endoscope is achieved using access point #2.

4) The desired sialendoscope is advanced over the stylet through the thyroid cartilage fenestration into Reinke's space followed by gentle infusion of saline, air, or gas to maximize visibility. A microendoscope also can be used for this purpose.

5) Injection or implantation of a substance can be performed through the created tunnel into the SLP in a similar fashion as GMT.

6) Surgical closure is accomplished similar to GMT.

Two scarred porcine larynges were evaluated rheologically 6 weeks following MERS-guided placement of HyStem-VF® (Biotime, Alameda), a hyaluronic acid-based hydrogel[35]. MERS-guided laryngoplasty using sialendoscopes yielded satisfactory biomaterial positioning in the short term and normalized rheologic tissue properties (elastic shear modulus, viscous modulus, and loss tangent) in the long term, contributing to proof of concept for MERS in the treatment of scar. Strengths of MERS include direct visualization of the SLP (and any accompanying pathology) and an ability to manipulate surgical instruments parallel to the vocal fold edge while maintaining an intact epithelium.

Future work has been proposed to explore the clinical utility of MERS for addressing scar, sulcus vocalis, and other intracordal processes. In addition, the development of micro-instruments that are small enough to pass through the working channel of a sialendoscope has been recommended. This includes microscissors, dissectors, and balloon dilators to access the SLP more effectively and to minimize the risk of penetrating the epithelium.

Conclusion

Treating vocal fold scar remains one of the greatest challenges in laryngology. When a decision has been made to treat vocal fold scar surgically, adherence to a few key surgical principles remains vital to achieving the ultimate goal of forming less symptomatic scar after surgery and improving mucosal wave. Restoration of mucosal wave is one important component of scar management. A variety of endoscopic and open surgical approaches has been described to aid in this endeavor, and success is achieved for many patients. In some cases, scar is too thick, too extensive, or too unstable for a vocal fold to benefit from the procedures described in this chapter. When these options have been exhausted or deemed inappropriate, more extensive procedures should be considered including surgery to replace the vocal fold edge with grafted tissue. Promising research on the effects of stem cells and growth factors to reduce scar formation suggests that they may be added to the list of available materials to treat vocal fold scar; and hopefully they will eventually render obsolete many of the techniques described in this chapter.

References

1. Hirano M. Morphological structure of the vocal cord as a vibrator and its variations. *Folia Phoniatr* 1974; 26:89–94.
2. Hansen JK and Thibeault SL. Current understanding and review of the literature: vocal fold scar. *J Voice* 2006; 20(1):110–120.
3. Thibeault SL, Gray SD, Bless DM, *et al.* Histologic and rheologic characterization of vocal fold scarring. *J Voice* 2002; 16(1):96–104.
4. Kass ES, Hillman RE, Zeitels SM. Vocal fold submucosal infusion technique in phonomicrosurgery. *Ann Otol Rhinol Laryngol* 1996; 105:341–347.
5. Burns JA, Friedman AD, Lutch MJ, Zeitels SM. Subepithelial vocal fold infusion: A useful diagnostic and therapeutic technique. *Ann Otol Rhinol Laryngol* 2012; 121(4):224–230.
6. Wang CT, Liao LJ, Cheng PW, *et al.* Intralesional steroid injection for benign vocal fold disorders: A systematic review and meta-analysis. *Laryngoscope* 2013; 123:197–203.
7. Benninger MS, Alessi D, Archer S, Bastian *et al.* Vocal fold scarring: Current concepts and management. *Otolaryngol Head Neck Surg* 1996; 115: 474–482.
8. Ford CN. Histologic study of injectable collagen in the canine larynx. *Laryngoscope* 1986; 96:1248–1257.
9. Ford CN, Bless DM, Loftus JM. Role of injectable collagen in the treatment of glottic insufficiency: a study of 199 patients. *Ann Otol Rhinol Laryngol* 1992; 101:23–47.
10. Ford CN, Bless DM. Collagen injection in the scarred vocal fold. *J Voice* 1987; 1:116–118
11. Sataloff RT. Vocal fold scar. In: Sataloff, RT. *Professional Voice: The Science and Art of Clinical Care* 3ed. San Diego, CA: Plural Publishing, Inc. 2005; pp 1309–1313.
12. Chhetri DK, Mendelsohn AH. Hyaluronic acid for the treatment of vocal fold scars. *Curr Opin Otolaryngol Head Neck Surg* 2010; 18:498–502.
13. Kwon TK and Buckmire R. Injection laryngoplasty for management of unilateral vocal fold paralysis. *Curr Opin Otolaryngol Head Neck Surg* 2004; 12: 538–542.
14. Lisi C, Hawkshaw MJ, Sataloff RT. Viscosity of materials for laryngeal injection: A review of current knowledge and clinical implications. *J Voice*. 2013; 27(1):119–123.
15. Ossoff RH, Koriwchak MJ, Netterville JL, Duncavage JA. Difficulties in endoscopic removal of Teflon granulomas of the vocal fold. *Ann Otol Rhinol Laryngol* 1993; 102(6):405–412.
16. Kasperbauer JL, Slavit DH, Maragos NE. Teflon granulomas and overinjection of Teflon: A therapeutic challenge for the otorhinolaryngologist. *Ann Otol Rhinol Laryngol* 1993; 102(10):748–751.

17. Chheda NN, Rosen CA, Belafsky PC, *et al*. Revision laryngeal surgery for the suboptimal injection of calcium hydroxylapatite. *Laryngoscope* 2008; 118(12):2260–3.

18. DeFatta RA, Chowdhury FR, Sataloff RT. Complications of injection laryngoplasty using calcium hydroxylapatite. *J Voice* 2012; 26(5):614–8.

19. Chan RW, Gray SD, Titze IR. The importance of hyaluronic acid in vocal fold biomechanics. *Otolaryngol Head Neck Surg* 2001; 124: 607–614.

20. Sataloff RT. Voice Surgery. In: Sataloff RT. *Professional Voice: The Science and Art of Clinical Care* 3ed San Diego, CA: Plural Publishing, Inc. 2005; pp 1161–1164.

21. Sataloff RT, Spiegel JR, Heuer RJ, *et al*. Laryngeal minimicroflap: a new technique and reassessment of the microflap saga. *J Voice* 1995; 9:198–204.

22. Sataloff RT, Spiegel JR, Hawkshaw M, *et al*. Autologous fat implantation for vocal fold scar: a preliminary report. *J Voice* 1997; 11(2):238–246.

23. Fleming DJ, McGuff S, Simpson CB. Comparison of microflap healing outcomes with traditional and microsuturing techniques: initial results in a canine model. *Ann Otol Rhinol Laryngol* 2001; 110:707–712.

24. Sataloff RT. Autologous fat implantation for vocal fold scar. *Curr Opin Otolaryngol Head Neck Surg* 2010; 18:503–506.

25. Neuenschwander MC, Sataloff RT, Abaza MM, *et al*. Management of vocal fold scar with autologous fat implantation: perceptual results. *J Voice* 2001; 15(2):295–304.

26. Pontes P, Behlau M. Treatment of sulcus vocalis: Auditory perceptual and acoustic analysis of the slicing mucosa surgical technique. *J Voice* 1993; 7: 365–376.

27. Pontes P, Behlau M. Sulcus mucosal slicing technique. *Curr Opin Otolaryngol Head Neck Surg* 2010; 18:512–520.

28. Sataloff RT. Voice surgery. In: Sataloff RT. *Professional Voice: The Science and Art of Clinical Care*, 3ed. San Diego, CA: Plural Publishing, Inc. 2005; pp 1206–1208.

29. Gray SD, Bielamowicz S, Titze I, *et al*. Experimental approaches to vocal fold alteration: introduction to the minithyrotomy. *Ann Otol Rhinol Laryngol* 1999; 108:1–9.

30. Mallur PS, Gartner-Schmidt J, Rosen C. Voice outcomes following the Gray minithyrotomy. *Ann Otol Rhinol Laryngol* 2012; 121:490–496.

31. Paniello RC, Sulica L, Khosla SM, Smith ME. Clinical experience with Gray's minithyrotomy procedure. *Ann Otol Rhinol Laryngol* 2008; 117:437–442.

32. Gunderson M, Bauer B, Glab RC, *et al*. Technical refinements to the minithyrotomy procedure. *J Voice* 2014; 28(4):501–507.

33. Dailey SH, Gunderson M, Chan R, *et al*. Local vascularized flaps for augmentation of Reinke's space. *Laryngoscope* 2011; 121(3):S37–S60.

34. Hoffman HT, Bock JM, Karnell LH, *et al*. Microendoscopy of Reinke's space. *Ann Otol Rhinol Laryngol* 2008; 117(7):510–514.

35. Bartlett RS, Hoffman HT, Dailey SH, *et al*. Restructuring the vocal fold lamina propria with endoscopic microdissection. *Laryngoscope* 2013; 123(11):2780–2786.

7

Management of sulcus vocalis

William E. Karle and Michael J. Pitman

Introduction

Sulcus vocalis is a derangement of the superficial lamina propria located along the free edge of the true vocal fold. It results in disturbance of vocal fold vibration and phonation. Although notoriously difficult to visualize on still light laryngoscopy, its effects often are seen on videostroboscopy, even when the sulcus itself is unidentifiable. Sulcus vocalis can cause severe dysphonia in a patient's voice including high-pitched and breathy dysphonia, phonatory breaks, vocal strain, decreased projection, and increased muscle tension[1-3]. It also may cause a bowed vocal fold configuration, mucosal stiffness, and glottic insufficiency[4]. These changes can be attributed to decreased pliability and decreased physical volume of the vocal fold. Frustratingly, there is no gold standard treatment for this disorder, which has led to the development of dozens of different surgical techniques. This chapter will cover the most widely used surgical methods for treating sulcus vocalis.

Sulcus vs scar

Although vocal fold scar and sulcus vocalis both represent abnormalities within the lamina propria, these two disorders should be thought of as separate entities. While vocal fold scar is primarily a deposition of abnormal tissue within the superficial lamina propria, sulcus is principally an absence of lamina propria with a strict configuration. It is important to note that abnormal lamina propria organization also occurs in sulcus vocalis, which has been shown to contain alterations of the collagenous and elastic fibers surrounding sulci[5]. Both vocal fold scar and sulcus often present with similar phonatory disturbances and share some of the same surgical options. Therefore, some of the management discussed here also will be covered in other chapters discussing the treatment of vocal fold scar.

Classification

The most widely used histopathologic classification system was created by Ford et al.[3], who divided sulcus vocalis into three groups. In type I, also referred to as physiologic sulcus, the overlying epithelium invaginates within the superficial layer of the lamina propria and does not adhere to the vocal ligament. This defect extends for the entire length of the musculomembranous vocal fold. As this type rarely affects the mucosal wave in any substantial way, it is often asymptomatic. However, these lesions may become physiologically significant if vocal loading is increased. As type I sulci are rarely treated surgically, this chapter will focus on types II and III.

Type II sulcus, also known as sulcus vergeture, extends through the superficial layer of the lamina propria, and epithelium is adherent to the vocal ligament. It often causes the vocal fold to appear spindle shaped, and the inferior and superior edges may either be flush to one another or present with a gap between them. Type III sulcus is defined as an epithelial invagination into the vocal ligament and/or vocalis muscle. This type of sulcus has the appearance of a pit, is more localized, and does not run along the entire length of the vocal fold. Type III are also more likely to be associated with severe underlying fibrosis and neovascularization of the true vocal fold[3].

Etiology and prevalence

It is likely that the etiologies of type II and type III sulci differ. Patients with type II sulci often note that their voices have been abnormal their entire life, while those with type III often have a more acute presentation. This supports researchers' belief that certain sulci may be congenital in origin, inherited in an autosomal dominant fashion[6]. Theories about why this anatomical defect may develop embryologically vary from the reappearance of a vestigial vocal fold to a defect in the 4th or 6th branchial arches[7]. Type II sulci are more often found bilaterally and in adult males[8,9]. Although still controversial, many laryngologists believe that sulcus vocalis type III occurs most commonly as a consequence of phonotrauma or inflammation. One convincing piece of evidence for this theory was provided by Nakayama *et al.* who showed an extremely high rate (48%) of sulcus vocalis in the contralateral vocal fold of patients with unilateral glottic cancer, suggesting its creation through chronic inflammation[10]. Others argue that type III sulcus vocalis is merely the result of a ruptured vocal cyst[11]. Disagreement also exists concerning the prevalence of sulcus vocalis, which is quoted in the literature as occurring in anywhere between 2.5–48% of the population[8,10,12]. This large discrepancy exists in part due to the examination of different populations and the particular definition used to designate what constitutes sulcus vocalis. In addition, due to the difficulty in visualizing a sulcus vocalis, the means of diagnosis, whether through cadaveric dissection, microlaryngoscopy, or flexible laryngoscopy also influences the prevalence reported (Figure 7.1).

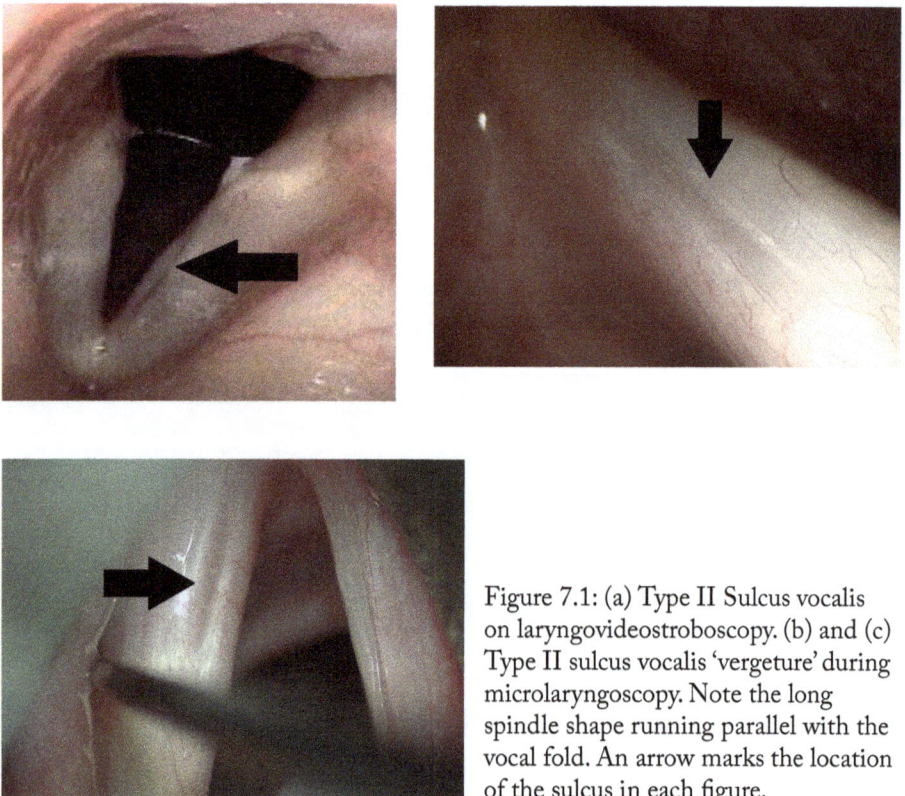

Figure 7.1: (a) Type II Sulcus vocalis on laryngovideostroboscopy. (b) and (c) Type II sulcus vocalis 'vergeture' during microlaryngoscopy. Note the long spindle shape running parallel with the vocal fold. An arrow marks the location of the sulcus in each figure.

Diagnosis

Diagnosing sulcus vocalis is quite difficult, and definitive identification often is not achieved until the patient undergoes microlaryngoscopy with palpation (Figure 7.2)[13]. As such, this disorder is often cited as being one of the most commonly missed glottic pathologies[14-16]. However, the appearance of vocal fold bowing leading to a spindle shaped glottis and the absence of a mucosal wave during phonation should cause the clinician to be suspicious of its presence[17].

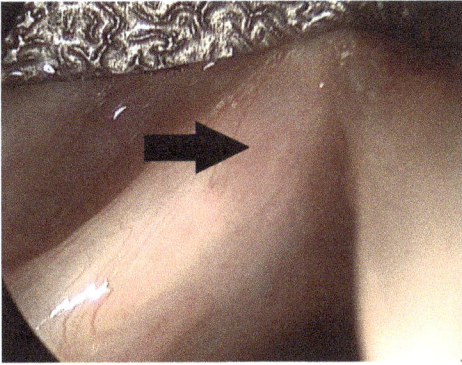

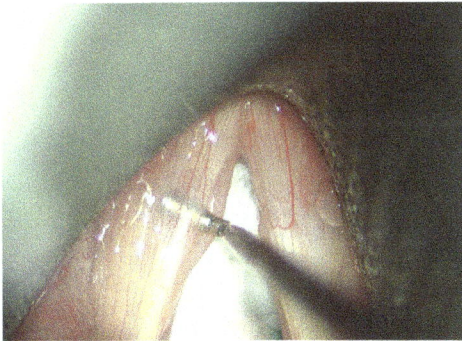

Figure 7.2: (a) A type III sulcus vocalis is very difficult to visualize during laryngovideostroboscopy and even during microlaryngoscopy without probing of the vocal fold. An arrow marks the location of the sulcus. (b) The sulcus identified with a blunt probe which details its position and depth.

The differential of disease processes causing this appearance is vast, ranging from presbylarynx to chronic laryngitis. In many patients with sulcus vocalis, there will also be a separate benign vocal fold lesion, the most common being polyps, cysts, and leukoplakia. It is also common to mistake what appears to be a cyst on videostroboscopy with what is actually a sulcus. During suspension laryngoscopy, palpation and meticulous examination must be performed for accurate diagnosis and surgical planning. It is also important that a thorough evaluation be performed on the patient before considering surgery. This includes a detailed voice assessment, videostroboscopy, high-speed video, and possibly discussion with other physicians and speech–language pathologists.

Current therapy

Conservative management should constitute the initial treatment for sulcus vocalis, regardless of the severity of dysphonia. This begins with optimization of a patient's voice by eliminating any aggravating factors. , which includes the treatment of laryngopharyngeal reflux (LPR), smoking cessation, control of allergies, and managing any other inflammatory disease affecting the larynx. It is important to recognize that sufficient positive results are more likely to occur if the patient is suffering from only mild-to-moderate dysphonia; and for patients with more severe dysphonia, surgery is often required.

Voice therapy also should be performed as part of conservative management prior to deciding on surgery. The goal of voice therapy is to optimize the patient's ability to phonate efficiently, in a non-traumatic manner. This may result in a voice that is satisfactory for the patient's needs. Once non-surgical treatment modalities have been attempted and substantial vocal impairment continues to exist, discussion of surgery should occur. If it has been determined that surgery will be required, voice therapy also can provide psychological preparation and education about proper expectations postoperatively. Voice therapy should then resume following a period of vocal rest after the procedure.

Although the surgical techniques available to a laryngologist for the correction of sulcus vocalis are numerous and varied, the majority share the same goals of either restoring the mucosal wave, correcting glottic incompetence, or both. In an attempt to restore the mucosal wave, surgeries have focused on replacing or repairing the superficial lamina propria or reorienting the vocal fold scar. In a different manner, glottic incompetence is corrected through augmentation of the vocal fold through either injection or framework surgery.

When bilateral sulci are present, the decision to perform bilateral simultaneous versus staged operations should take into consideration how important the use of voice is to the patient's profession, degree of vocal dysfunction, and the expertise of the surgeon. It is the senior author's (MJP) recommendation that bilateral sulci may be treated safely during the same operation in selected cases. Sulcus vocalis occurring on both vocal folds is quite common, and several studies have noted its prevalence as occurring in >50% of surgical patients[18].

Surgical treatment of sulcus vocalis

There are no strict contraindications to the surgical treatment of sulcus vocalis, but a surgeon would be wise to act conservatively if a patient has untreated laryngitis due to other medical pathologies or active rheumatologic disease. Perhaps the most important aspect of preoperative care is the management of realistic expectations. Restoration of a normal voice may occur, but is not likely, and is not a reasonable expectation. The goals are to improve the voice so that it is fuller, louder, clearer, more stable, requiring less strain, experiencing less fatigue, and becoming more reliable with fewer exacerbations of dysphonia.

Currently there are no defined guidelines for distinguishing which patients are more likely to achieve success from surgical intervention. Unfortunately, the majority of published studies evaluating surgery for sulcus vocalis have been limited to a single institution and are retrospective in design. To complicate matters, one of the few prospective multi-arm studies looking at treatment of sulcus vocalis found no statistical difference in surgical success between type I laryngoplasty, injection laryngoplasty, and temporalis fascia graft[19]. Consequently, there is still much debate about which specific surgery should be recommended for these patients. Surgery is indicated generally for patients who have failed conservative therapy and are motivated to undergo further intervention due to the impact of dysphonia on their quality of life. Patients must have reasonable expectations as well as understand and be willing to accept the risks of the chosen intervention.

The surgeon should make every effort to achieve full visualization of the glottis using direct microlaryngoscopy for optimal evaluation and surgical treatment of sulcus vocalis. If adequate visualization is not possible, the surgeon may be limited to performing a type I laryngoplasty or transcervical procedure. Another question that must also be answered by the surgeon during surgical planning is whether to use an implantable graft and, if so, whether it should be autologous, thus requiring a harvest site. It is also important to understand whether the surgery proposed is designed as a temporary trial measure or a more permanent solution

Many surgical approaches for the treatment of sulcus vocalis are performed using suspension microlaryngoscopy. Although varied in technique, these surgeries all start with the same steps. Unless otherwise mentioned, the patient usually should be sedated with general anesthesia with respiration maintained using either jet-ventilation or endotracheal intubation.

Using an appropriate large bore laryngoscope for optimal glottic visualization, close inspection and palpation of the vocal folds should be performed using straight and angled telescopes in order to determine the depth and configuration of the sulcus vocalis as well as identifying any other glottic lesions. A subepithelial infusion of saline with or without 1:10,000 epinephrine will aid in delineation of the sulcus, as it will remain adherent to the underlying tissue while the surrounding healthy tissue elevates. If a separate glottic lesion is identified, it is often removed during the same operation, prior to treatment of the sulcus vocalis. Regardless of the method chosen, close attention should be paid to sparing the normal mucosa adjacent to the anterior commissure to avoid formation of a glottic web. If a bilateral procedure is planned and the result of the first side is suboptimal, the procedure should be staged. Although decided on a case by case basis, unless specific untoward comorbidities exist, all procedures described are ambulatory surgeries.

Microflap elevation with excision

The goal of this operation is to remove the entire epithelial lining of the sulcus, including any adherent abnormal fibrous tissue. This is achieved using a subepithelial dissection similar to a microflap. This procedure's only aim is to improve mucosal mobility and it does not attempt to correct any glottic insufficiency caused by the absent superficial lamina propria. Although described here using cold steel, this method can also be performed using a laser, which is described later in this chapter.

Technique

The mucosa is incised using a curved sickle knife in the anterior to posterior direction along the vocal fold's superior face adjacent to the sulcus[20]. A blunt probe or elevator is then used to dissect within the subepithelial plane and release the adherent sulcus. Medial retraction of the epithelium exposes the plane between the epithelium and underlying tissue. This can be performed with forceps or microsuction with a velvet eye. Though more difficult to use, the velvet eye suction has the benefit of suctioning pooling fluids as well as decreasing the risk of tearing the epithelium. If the epithelium is not easily dissected using this method, microscissors can be used with close attention paid to avoiding perforation.

Once the sulcus has been detached completely from the underlying tissue, a second linear incision is made just inferior to the sulcus, parallel to the free edge of the vocal fold. The most anterior and posterior attachments to normal mucosa should then be cut and the sulcus removed en bloc. As little healthy mucosa possible should be taken when making each incision. Depending on the size of the resection, a millimeter or two of healthy mucosa often requires undermining along either edge to allow a tension-free closure over the gap that has been created. Interrupted 6-0 or 7-0 absorbable sutures placed within 1 mm of the wound edge may be used for closure and reapproximation of the wound edges.

Microflap elevation without excision

This technique is rarely used but has benefits as one of the more conservative approaches for treatment of sulcus vocalis with minimal risk. In contrast to sulcus excision, the surgeon preserves potentially useful epithelium and minimizes the risks of increased scarring and greater glottal insufficiency due to deeper tissue resection or lateral scar retraction. The goal of this method is to redrape the epithelium in a more natural position. It is also believed that the tissue healing and repair might result in a more pliable cover.

Technique

This technique begins in the same manner described above, but once the sulcus is detached from the underlying vocal ligament and redraped, the procedure has been completed. Using this technique, only the first mucosal incision is made as compared to the two incisions required for excision. Attempts should be made to free all aspects of the sulcus epithelium from the underlying vocal ligament and muscle. If multiple perforations or tears have occurred during this method and tissue viability is questioned, proceeding with excision of the sulcus should be reconsidered.

Lasers

The 585-nm pulsed dye laser (PDL)[21], 532-nm KTP laser[22], and 10.6 μm CO_2 laser[18] have all been described for treatment of sulcus vocalis. The CO_2 laser is used as a dissection tool, while the KTP and PDL lasers are used to stimulate tissue remodeling as based on results in the treatment of hypertrophic scarring and scarring from acne excoriee[23]. A CO_2 laser may be used for any maneuver described using cold dissection with the same principles in mind. During laser use, expert care must be taken to avoid inadvertent injury to the surrounding tissues by excess diffusion of heat. Supporters of this technology believe that the laser provides a more controlled and precise dissection, allowing the surgeon to more easily stay in the correct plane[18]. For further details see Chapter 9: Lasers.

Technique for photoangiolytic glottoplasty

KTP and PDL lasers are used commonly in the office and operating room for the treatment of several types of benign lesions. In the patient with sulcus vocalis, general anesthesia should be considered, as significant manipulation of the vocal fold is required for adequate sulcus exposure. This technique is generally better for type II sulcus as the deep invagination of a type III sulcus would not be expected to improve physiologically with this treatment.

Improvement in phonation has been reported after treatment of vocal fold scar and sulcus vocalis with the PDL[21,24]. As the KTP laser has become more popular, it has replaced the PDL for such treatment in many centers. No outcomes have been reported for the treatment of sulcus vocalis with a KTP laser.

Typically the PDL laser will be set at 0.75 Joules per pulse and the KTP at approximately 35 W and 15 ms, although some surgeons use lower settings. Ultimately the endpoint of treatment is epithelial blanching, described as a type I treatment.[25]

Mucosal slicing technique

This technique was designed by Pontes and Behlau for sulcus patients who have an absent mucosal wave and large glottic chink[26,27]. The purpose of this procedure is to interrupt the tension lines created by the sulci, while also decreasing the glottic gap and repairing the mucosal wave. It is important to note that this technique involves many more mucosal incisions than any other proposed surgical method. Therefore, there exists a risk of fibrosis during wound healing. Thin mucosal adhesions are sometimes seen two weeks postoperatively and should be released in the office or OR, and a substantial risk of granuloma formation also exists. As these granulomas often undergo spontaneous remission, they should be treated surgically only if they become enlarged or continue to be present for a prolonged time postop. It is also very important that the patient understands that they risk experiencing severe dysphonia for three to four months postoperatively. Due to these risks and the questionable benefit of the procedure, it is has mostly fallen out of favor.

Technique

This procedure begins with a longitudinal (anterior–posterior) mucosal incision made lateral to the free edge of the vocal fold using a straight or curved sickle knife. The incision should be made as close to the laryngeal ventricle as possible and at least 3 mm lateral to the sulcus. Next, the mucosa and underlying vocal ligament located medial to the incision are elevated using a blunt instrument. This newly created flap should extend under and approximately 3 mm past the sulcus. The flap should be at least 2 mm in depth and may extend as deep as the thyroarytenoid muscle in order to preserve sufficient blood supply to the flap. Following this, three to five "counter" incisions are made extending perpendicularly from the initial incision and continuing through the inferior lip of the sulcus, producing either three or four inferiorly based flaps. These incisions can be made using micro scissors and should vary in length to cause a difference in height between the mucosal flaps. If done correctly, the flaps should lie in appropriate opposition without the need for manipulation, and accordingly the use of sutures or glue is discouraged. If a sulcus is present bilaterally, it has been recommended that both be treated during the same operation, although this recommendation is controversial and not based on evidence.

Autologous graft implantation

To date, the most promising reconstructive techniques for sulcus vocalis involve the insertion of biologic materials into the obliterated Reinke's space. These can either be autologous or heterologous. Several different materials have been investigated, with the majority of autologous materials involving either fat or fascia. All grafts are likely to experience some reabsorption, although the degree to which this happens is usually less with autologous materials[28]. Regardless of the material selected, one of the potential complications involves extrusion from the vocal fold. If the partial extrusion occurs, a granuloma will often form at the site. Because of this possibility, some surgeons recommend that 7-0 interrupted suture is used to approximate the mucosal edges of the incision and fibrin glue be used to seal it[29]. Details of a non-suture technique are discussed in Chapter 6 on epithelium freeing techniques.

Autologous fat

Fat grafts via injection augmentation of the vocal fold are typically used for the treatment of glottal insufficiency in sulcus vocalis. Previously, placement of fat into the obliterated Reinke's space had been used rarely due to the difficulty in handling, placing and securing the graft.[30] However, they are now used more often, employing the technique described in Chapter 6. The use of autologous adipose grafts was first developed in 1991 to avoid a foreign body reaction, which is possible with bovine collagen.[31] Similar to collagen, transplanted fat within the vocal folds also experiences significant postoperative reabsorption, as noted in the first report of fat injection.[32] Submucosally implanted fat was introduced in 1997 and may resorb less than injected fat.[33] This adipose tissue is implanted during microlaryngoscopy, following undermining of the sulcus.

It is important to place as much adipose tissue within the vocal fold as possible, as anywhere between 40–50% of it will be reabsorbed within a year.[30] As with all implant techniques, extravasation of the implanted graft is one of the most likely post-op complications. This risk is mitigated when adipose tissue is inserted with a transoral injection into the vocal fold using an 18 gauge needle. The injection can either be placed within the vocal ligament or in a submucosal plane. By using a fat injection alone there is no need for a mucosal incision. However, fat distribution and lysis of scar adhesions are more limited with this technique than with the special flap technique described elsewhere and in Chapter 5. Its use through injection also mandates that the fat be able to pass through a syringe. The senior author centrifuges the fat for this procedure, while others wash the fat with saline.

Autologous fat graft technique

The procedure should begin with microflap elevation of the sulcus to ensure flap integrity prior to fat harvest. Care should be taken to avoid perforation during elevation, which could lead to fat extravasation. The donor site is often the subcutaneous tissue in the posterior aspect of the lobule, umbilicus, or axilla. The graft should be cleaned of any adherent skin follicles or dermis that may have been mistakenly removed with the graft. There are multiple ways for preparing the fat after harvest. One typical procedure involves washing the fat with copious amounts of saline and then storing it in saline.[30]

The adipose tissue may be inserted within the pocket and the mucosal incision closed by using three or four mucosal sutures; however, sutures can be avoided using the self-closing trap door flap technique.[33,34] Fibrin glue should then be applied to seal the incision and add an extra level of protection against extravasation. Further palpation or manipulation of the vocal folds should be done using only a minimal amount of pressure to ensure the implant will not extravasate.

Autologous fascia

Autologous transplantation of fascia into the vocal fold (ATFV) using temporalis fascia within Reinke's space was introduced in 1999 by Tsunoda.[35] Although the outcome data for ATFV are scarce, as it is for all treatments of sulcus vocalis, this method currently appears to be one of the most promising techniques. Studies of ATFV have shown restoration of the mucosal wave and improvement of glottal closure within one year of this procedure for patients with sulcus vocalis.[28] Using the GRBAS (grade, roughness, breathiness, asthenia, strain) rating scale other studies have shown significant improvement overall in all subscales except breathiness.[29] The most common complication encountered for ATFV is extrusion or herniation,[28] which may lead to granuloma formation. It is unclear whether the restoration of the mucosal wave and glottal closure is due to the fascia itself, or stimulated wound healing activity resulting in tissue remodeling.[28] Although no exact time range can be cited, most authors agree that the vocal recovery from this surgery is often longer than other treatments for sulcus vocalis, taking 3 –6 months, and this should be discussed with the patient preoperatively.

ATFV technique

This procedure begins with an incision at the superior edge of the sulcus and careful elevation of the epithelium overlying the sulcus vocalis. Care is taken to keep the flap intact; and, if necessary, a small amount of muscle may be elevated with the flap. The pocket should span beyond the anterior, posterior, and inferior edges of the sulcus so that the graft can overlap the abnormal area. Once the integrity of the flap is ensured, the temporalis fascia is harvested in the standard fashion used for a tympanoplasty, obtaining a 1cm x 1cm graft. A piece of sterilized ruler is cut as a template and inserted into the pocket. The piece of ruler is trimmed until it can fill the entire pocket lying flat without undue mucosal tension. Using this template, the temporalis fascia is then trimmed to the identical size.

If the patient has severe glottic incompetence, greater bulk can be achieved by pressing one layer of temporalis onto another before insertion, which will add greater volume. This is more difficult and may be unnecessary considering the theory of fibroblast and other healing factors stimulation as a primary reason for success of the surgery. To prevent rapid re-expansion of the graft, the pocket should first be dried using a small pledget or cotton tip. Using straight alligator tissue forceps, the temporalis fascia is inserted into the vocal fold pocket and its position adjusted using a blunt needle (Figure 7.3). When suturing the incision closed, care must be taken to only pass the needle through the epithelium, avoiding the underlying transplanted graft. If the graft is pierced by the needle, it with will twist up as the suture is pulled through, displacing the graft and possibly causing a partial extrusion through the needle puncture (Figure 7.4). After the suture approximates the mucosal edges, fibrin glue may be used to seal the length of incision and decrease the likelihood of graft herniation.

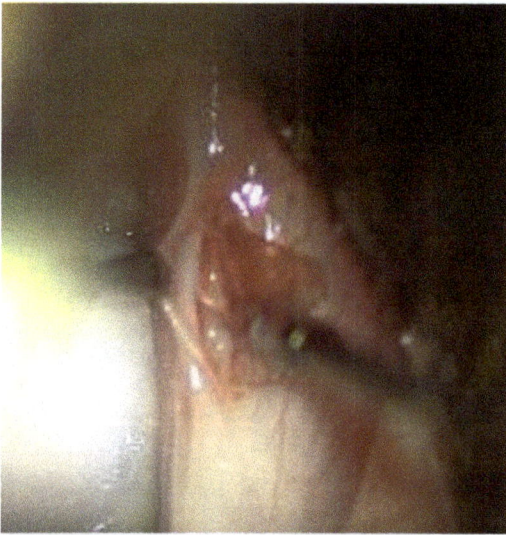

Figure 7.3: Insertion of the temporalis fascia graft into the mucosal pocket created within the vocal fold.

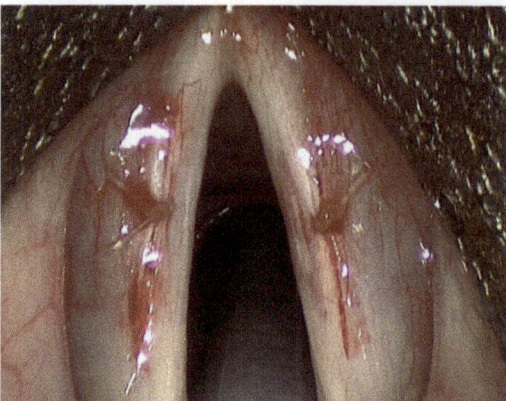

Figure 7.4: Reapproximation of the mucosal free edges following the placement of temporalis fascia for the treatment of bilateral vocal fold sulci. Subsequently fibrin glue is placed over the incision to prevent graft herniation.

Steroid injection

Steroid injection for the treatment of vocal fold scar is often used due to its low risk profile and anecdotal success. Although potentially useful, only a few studies have demonstrated significant positive functional outcomes, and more research is needed.[36] Steroid injections have been used as solitary treatment, or following completion of any number of surgical procedures. Steroids are injected into the surgical field or directly into the scar and surrounding region of the superficial lamina propria. They are used for both their anti-inflammatory and immune modulating properties, and as hydrodissection to lyse soft adhesions. Aside from the obvious anti-inflammatory benefits, steroids are thought to work by decreasing collagen synthesis and increasing its degradation.[37,38] The most commonly used steroids for this procedure are methylprednisolone 40mg/ml, triamcinolone acetonide, and dexamethasone.[36,39]

Injection augmentation

The use of injectable augmentation for the correction of sulcus vocalis was one of the first surgical techniques developed. This began with the injection of paraffin by Brünings in 1911; however, over time more biologically inert substances have taken its place. Unlike the previously described surgeries for sulcus vocalis, injections can be performed in the clinic setting. The route by which the needle is inserted into the true vocal fold is either percutaneous or transorally. If transoral injection is to be done in the office, a curved needle and fiberoptic laryngoscope should be used, while in the operating room, direct laryngoscopy and a straight needle are employed. If done percutaneously, the injection can be performed under laryngoscopic guidance through the cricothyroid membrane, thyrohyoid membrane, or thyroid cartilage (translaryngeal); however, some surgeons prefer to perform this injection blindly.

The main goal of these procedures is to add volume to the true vocal fold and decrease glottic incompetence. Injections have been shown to work well for glottic defects under 3mm, whereas larger deficits are more often corrected using laryngeal framework surgery.[40] The most common complication from injections is extravasation. Other potential complications from injection include inflammatory reaction, bleeding from the injection site, infection, and vocal strain. A rare but unfortunate side effect may occur if the injection is placed into the superficial lamina propria, causing vocal fold stiffness or scar formation.

The different materials used for injection can be grouped into either short or long acting treatments. Although all injectable material is at risk for reabsorption, those classified as short acting often last for only three to six months (or less). Due to reabsorption, overinjection by approximately 15–30% is recommended commonly. Although the injection can be done as a standalone procedure, some believe more successful results can be obtained if it is combined with one of the above procedures performed on the vocal fold cover.[41] This would necessitate that the procedure be done under general anesthesia. Thus, for some patients, doing the injection alone may be preferred. Temporary injections performed in the office are also often done as a therapeutic trial to determine the chance of improvement before committing to a more durable injection or permanent type I laryngoplasty.

Injection technique

As discussed, prior to injection under general anesthesia, the option exists to perform surgery on the sulcus vocalis and vocal fold cover. The injection augmentation is performed identically to injection augmentation for vocal fold paralysis and vocal fold atrophy. The injection material should be placed into the lateral aspect of the body of the vocal fold. Typically, the injection is performed at the junction of the anterior and mid third of the vocal fold, lateral to the presumed striking zone, or further posteriorly. The amount injected will vary depending on the degree of glottic incompetence and the properties of the injectable chosen. As previously mentioned, most injections should receive a 15–30% overcorrection in volume, excluding the use of autologous fat. For autologous fat, doubling the amount of injection is recommended to account for the rapid partial reabsorption that often occurs. In addition, fibrin glue may be used to close the puncture hole made by the larger bore needle associated with autologous fat injection. In-office injections can be performed through the cricothyroid membrane, thyrohyoid membrane, or thyroid cartilage. Their specific techniques are described elsewhere.[42]

Temporary acting products

Collagen Products – Autologous, AlloDerm™ (LifeCell Corporation, Branchburg, NJ), Cymetra™ (LifeCell Corporation, Branchburg, NJ), Zyplast™ (Allergan, Irvine, CA)

Originally developed by Ford *et al*,[43] bovine collagen was described first in 1984 as a method of adding vocal fold bulk to decrease the risk of foreign body reaction, as compared to the allogenic materials used at that time. However, further research has shown that this treatment may cause allergic reactions, delayed systemic hypersensitivity, and vocal fold fibrosis in certain patients.[44] Theoretically, the risk of transmitting bovine spongiform encephalopathy also exists. Another detriment of using this material is the necessity of pre-operative skin testing to bovine allergens. Several studies have also shown that bovine collagen only remains within the vocal fold for two to six months before reabsorption.[18]

Acellular human cadaveric collagen matrices and autologous collagen have largely replaced bovine collagen. Both eliminate the risk of an allergic reaction, and the autologous collagen also eliminates the risk of disease transmission. Of these, the autologous collagen has the longest half-life. However, a disadvantage of using autologous collagen is the necessity of a skin donor site, which usually requires being taken from the lower abdomen below the bikini line. Autologous collagen also necessitates a staged procedure, with the first procedure involving skin harvesting and production of injectable collagen, before returning to the operating room for injection at some future date. The main goal of collagen injections is to add sufficient bulk to decrease glottic incompetence. However, the use of collagen also has been shown to assist in recovery of the mucosal wave, which may return as early as one month post-operatively.

Hyaluronic acid gel – Restylane™ (Galderma, Fort Worth, TX), Hylaform™ (Genzyme, Cambridge, MA)

Hyaluronic acid is an anionic, nonsulfated glycosaminoglycan found in most types of connective tissue within the body, with an especially high level within the extracellular matrix of the superficial lamina propria. Originally designed for the treatment of rhytids, crosslinked hyaluronic acid forms an injectable viscous substance. Recent research has suggested that hyaluronic acid is a key component for the fluidity of the superficial lamina propria (SLP). For this reason, hyaluronic acid is now an option for vocal fold injection. Research has shown also that these injections often last four to nine months within the true vocal fold, but benefits have been demonstrated for up to one year post-operatively.[45]

Carboxymethylcellulose – Prolaryn Gel® (Merz, Raleigh, NC)

Carboxymethylcellulose (CMC) augmentation usually lasts between two to three months before reabsorption.[46] Although positive results have been demonstrated in patients with immobility or hypomobility of the true vocal folds, outcomes have been more modest in patients with sulcus vocalis or scar.[47] One of the disadvantages of this product is the risk of mild chronic inflammatory changes and foreign body reactions. If these reactions are present, there is no evidence that they will lead to significant or chronic granuloma formation.[48]

Durable acting products

Calcium Hydroxylapatite – Prolaryn Plus® (Merz, Raleigh, NC)

This injectable contains microspheres of calcium hydroxylapatite within a gel carrier. Evidence indicates that it lasts approximately 19 months within the body.[49] When used for glottal insufficiency, 64% of patients will eventually lose any positive results of the procedure, with the average duration of benefit lasting approximately 18 months.[49] Due to the properties of calcium hydroxylapatite, the injection must be accurate, deep, and lateral in the thyroarytenoid muscle. Inaccurate injections or migration of the material can lead to significant complications such as granulomas and vocal fold vibration disturbance resulting in severe dysphonia.[50] Due to this, in-office injection is discouraged because of the inherent decrease in accuracy when compared to injection under general anesthesia.

Autologous fat

See previous section 'Autologous graft implantation.'

Gray's minithyrotomy

Originally described by Gray *et al* in 1999,[51] using Gray's minithyrotomy approach, varying materials (ex: allograft and fascia) can be implanted into the subepithelial plane of the true vocal fold using an external incision and a small defect created within the thyroid cartilage. The major advantage of this approach is the avoidance of a mucosal incision or mucosal perforation with an injection needle. This procedure is indicated for patients with either sulcus vocalis or vocal fold scar and is generally used only for patients with more severe disease. Designed primarily for increasing the mucosal wave, it has less impact on glottic competence due to the limited volume which may be inserted into the vocal fold using the method in Gray's classic description. Imaginative in design, its results have been mixed to date, with a significant risk of long term worsened phonation due to this procedure.[52]

Gray's minithyrotomy technique

Endotracheal intubation and general anesthesia are used commonly. Due to the profound edema that may occur, it is recommended that 10mg of decadron be injected intravenously immediately prior to the start of the procedure. A large bore laryngoscope is used for suspension laryngoscopy and subsequent palpation and visualization using a zero or thirty degree endoscope. This scope should be held by an assistant while a 3cm horizontal incision is made over the inferior 1/3 of the thyroid cartilage. Dissection proceeds down to the strap muscles and the median raphe is incised allowing lateral retraction of the straps. The thyroid cartilage should be cleaned of any adherent tissue using a Kitner or similar dissector, sharp curved scissors, or scalpel.

A 22 gauge needle is passed through the midline of the thyroid cartilage into the laryngeal lumen to locate the exact level of the anterior commissure. Using a #15 blade, a perichondrial incision is made along the midline of the thyroid cartilage, followed by perichondrial elevation using a freer. Once a 1cm x 1cm square of perichondrium has been elevated, a power drill using a 3mm cutting burr is placed 3mm lateral to the midline of the anterior commissure. The drill should be orientated directly horizontal to the vocal fold, aiming straight down at the underlying table (which may be tilted rather than parallel to the floor if the head and head piece have been extended). Drilling should cease once through the cartilage, but prior to perforation of the inner perichondrium. A 'give' should be felt once at the appropriate level. A mastoid curette can be used to remove any remaining cartilage overlying the perichondrium. Using a small knife, an incision is made through the inner perichondrium. Blunt dissection should then proceed within the subepithelial plane while it is visualized using the endoscope. Various otologic instruments can be used to continue the dissection until the entire vibratory edge of the membranous vocal fold is undermined. At this point, the patient is ready for graft placement.

The most commonly used graft material for this procedure is autologous fat; however, several other materials such as AlloDerm™ and fascia have been described. If using autologous fat, the harvest can often occur from the subcutaneous tissue encountered during dissection. For this reason, dissection should be performed without electrocautery. Usually 1cc of fat is sufficient for each vocal fold.

The fat can be placed as a single graft or centrifuged and injected using an angiocatheter, while other surgeons prefer to harvest it through a large (8–10mm) liposuction cannula and deliver it through a Brünings syringe. Regardless of the material, it is important that it be distributed evenly lengthwise along the vocal fold. This can be aided by the assistant working through the laryngoscope, using a long blunt instrument massaging the edge of the vocal fold. Once in adequate position, the thyroid cartilage burr holes are closed with bone wax, followed by closure of the soft tissue in standard fashion.

Medialization laryngoplasty

Medialization laryngoplasty, also referred to as Isshiki type I thyroplasty, is a laryngeal framework surgery commonly used for patients with glottic incompetence. This technique has long been used for patients suffering from several different vocal fold disorders, including but not limited to vocal fold paralysis, vocal fold scar, cancer defects, and sulcus vocalis. These surgeries have been shown to have substantial success in correcting glottic incompetence. In addition, medialization laryngoplasty does not address the absence of the mucosal wave. The implants used within the vocal fold include Silastic®, Gore-tex®, hydroxylapatite, and other pre-fashioned materials. Strap muscle transposition has also been used as an autologous option.[53] The details of these procedures are found in Chapter 5: Medialization procedures.

Growth factors

Growth factors are endogenous substances that have the ability to stimulate cell growth, healing, proliferation, migration, and differentiation. Theoretically, exogenously produced growth factors should cause the same outcomes when injected into the targeted tissue. In 2008, Hirano *et al* were the first to publish the use of injectable growth factor within the human vocal fold.[54] To date, the only growth factor that has been investigated in humans as a potential treatment for sulcus vocalis is the basic fibroblast growth factor (bFGF).[55] Delivered either as an injection or impregnated on a gelatin sponge implanted in Reinke's space, the results have been promising. Although only a small sample size from a single site has been reported to date, this mode of treatment could hold great promise in coming years. Before a recommendation can be made, further studies with longer follow-up must be performed. For more details see Chapter 10: Tissue engineering.

Post-operative care

Post-operative care varies from surgeon to surgeon; however, basic principles are presented here. Regardless of the surgical technique, strict vocal rest is recommended post-operatively for operations on the vibratory edge of the vocal fold. Voice rest may vary from 2–14 days but is generally in line with the surgeon's practice for a typical microflap phonosurgery. Voice rest after vocal fold injections is variable and again similar to that of a typical injection for vocal fold augmentation. Once the patient is allowed to speak, he/she should restart voice therapy. The typical post-operative voice therapy regimen involves between 5–6 sessions, occurring once a week (details in Chapter 4). However, these patients may require longer periods of voice therapy because of the slow healing process, with structural changes occurring in many cases for a year. The use of antibiotics for these procedures is controversial, and no clear evidence exists for their use. If used, no more than five days of antibiotics post-operatively are prescribed for most patients. Although commonly used in the perioperative period, there also exists no evidence for the use of steroids after surgery.

The patient should be seen for their first post-operative visit approximately one week following surgery, at which point videostroboscopy may be performed. After the initial visit, the patient is typically seen intermittently, at least 3–4 times over the following year, with videostroboscopic examination usually performed at each visit. The duration until optimal vocal improvement is dependent on the type of surgery and patient response, and while it may be just a few weeks for vocal fold injection, it may take six to twelve months for ATFV and fat implantation.

Conclusion

Although a large armamentarium of materials and techniques exists for the treatment of sulcus vocalis, the majority of results are inconsistent at best. The number of options is in and of itself indicative of the lack of a consistently successful surgery. While ATVF and fat implantation appear to have good, consistent results, recovery is prolonged. The early success with growth factors also holds hope for advances in this area; however, continued research and surgical innovation are needed for further progress.

References

1. Welham NV, Dailey SH, Ford CN, Bless DM. Voice handicap evaluation of patients with pathologic sulcus vocalis. *Ann Otol Rhinol Laryngol* 2007; 116(6):411–417.
2. Hirano M, Yoshida T, Tanaka S, Hibi S. Sulcus vocalis: functional aspects. *Ann Otol Rhinol Laryngol* 1990; 99(9 Pt 1):679–683.
3. Ford CN, Inagi K, Khidr A, *et al*. Sulcus vocalis: a rational analytical approach to diagnosis and management. *Ann Otol Rhinol Laryngol.* Mar 1996; 105(3):189–200.
4. Thibeault SL, Gray SD, Bless DM, *et al*. Histologic and rheologic characterization of vocal fold scarring. *J Voice* 2002; 16(1):96–104.
5. Sato K, Hirano M. Electron microscopic investigation of sulcus vocalis. *Ann Otol Rhinol Laryngol* 1998; 107(1):56–60.
6. Martins RH, Goncalves TM, Neves DS, *et al*. Sulcus vocalis: evidence for autosomal dominant inheritance. *Genet Mol Res* 2011; 10(4):3163–3168.
7. Bouchayer M, Cornut G, Witzig E, *et al*. Epidermoid cysts, sulci, and mucosal bridges of the true vocal cord: a report of 157 cases. *Laryngoscope* 1985; 95(9 Pt 1):1087–1094.
8. Sunter AV, Yigit O, Huq GE, *et al*. Histopathological characteristics of sulcus vocalis. *Otolaryngol Head Neck Surg* 2011; 145(2):264–269.
9. Zhukhovitskaya A, Battaglia D, Khosla SM, *et al*. Gender and age in benign vocal fold lesions. *Laryngoscope* 2015; 125(1):191–196.
10. Nakayama M, Ford CN, Brandenburg JH, Bless DM. Sulcus vocalis in laryngeal cancer: a histopathologic study *Laryngoscope* 1994; 104(1 Pt 1):16–24.
11. Watson GJ, Jones PH. Videographic documentation of an open cyst converting into a sulcus vocalis. *J Voice* Sep 2011; 25(5):e221–222.
12. Hsiung MW, Woo P, Wang HW, Su WY. A clinical classification and histopathological study of sulcus vocalis. *Eur Arch Otorhinolaryngol* 2000; 257(8):466–468.
13. Giovanni A, Chanteret C, Lagier A. Sulcus vocalis: a review. *Eur Arch Otorhinolaryngol* 2007; 264(4):337–344.
14. Poels PJ, de Jong FI, Schutte HK. Consistency of the preoperative and intraoperative diagnosis of benign vocal fold lesions. *J Voice* 2003; 17(3):425–433.

15. Dailey SH, Spanou K, Zeitels SM. The evaluation of benign glottic lesions: rigid telescopic stroboscopy versus suspension microlaryngoscopy. *J Voice* 2007; 21(1):112–118.

16. Akbulut S, Altintas H, Oguz H. Videolaryngostroboscopy versus microlaryngoscopy for the diagnosis of benign vocal cord lesions: a prospective clinical study. *Eur Arch Otorhinolaryngol* 2015;272(1):131–136.

17. Lim JY, Kim J, Choi SH, *et al*. Sulcus configurations of vocal folds during phonation. *Acta oto-laryngologica* 2009; 129(10):1127–1135.

18. Remacle M, Lawson G, Degols JC, *et al*. Microsurgery of sulcus vergeture with carbon dioxide laser and injectable collagen. *Ann Otol Rhino Laryngol* 2000; 109(2):141–148.

19. Welham NV, Choi SH, Dailey SH, *et al*. Prospective multi-arm evaluation of surgical treatments for vocal fold scar and pathologic sulcus vocalis. *Laryngoscope* 2011; 121(6):1252–1260.

20. Yilmaz T. Sulcus vocalis: excision, primary suture and medialization laryngoplasty: personal experience with 44 cases. *Eur Arch Otorhinolaryngol* 2012; 269(11):2381–2389.

21. Hwang CS, Lee HJ, Ha JG, *et al*. Use of pulsed dye laser in the treatment of sulcus vocalis. *Otolaryngol Head Neck Surg* 2013; 148(5):804–809.

22. Hosokawa K, Watanabe Y, Imai T, *et al*. New operation for sulcus vocalis: laser vaporization of the sulcus with fat injection. *Nihon Jibiinkoka Gakkai kaiho* 2007; 110(8):581–585.

23. Lack EB, Rachel JD. Resolution of retracted scar after 585-nm pulse dye laser surgery. *J Cosmet Laser* Nov 2004; 6(3):149–151.

24. Mortensen MM, Woo P, Ivey C, *et al*. The use of the pulse dye laser in the treatment of vocal fold scar: a preliminary study. *Laryngoscope* 2008; 118(10):1884–1888.

25. Mallur PS, Johns MM, III, Amin MR, Rosen CA. Proposed classification system for reporting 532-nm pulsed potassium titanyl phosphate laser treatment effects on vocal fold lesions. *Laryngoscope* 2014; 124(5):1170–1175.

26. Pontes P, Behlau M. Sulcus mucosal slicing technique. *Curr Opin Otolaryngol Head Neck Surg* Dec 2010; 18(6):512–520.

27. Pontes P, Behlau M. Treatment of sulcus vocalis: auditory perceptual and acoustical analysis of the slicing mucosa surgical technique. *J Voice* 1993; 7(4):365–376.

28. Tsunoda K, Kondou K, Kaga K, *et al*. Autologous transplantation of fascia into the vocal fold: long-term result of type-1 transplantation and the future. *Laryngoscope* 2005; 115(12 Pt 2 Suppl 108):1–10.

29. Pitman MJ, Rubino SM, Cooper AL. Temporalis fascia transplant for vocal fold scar and sulcus vocalis. *Laryngoscope* 2014; 124(7):1653–1658.

30. Pinto JA, da Silva Freitas ML, Carpes AF, *et al*. Autologous grafts for treatment of vocal sulcus and atrophy. *Otolaryngol Head Neck Surg* 2007; 137(5):785–791.

31. Mikaelian DO, Lowry LD, Sataloff RT. Lipoinjection for unilateral vocal cord paralysis. *Laryngoscope* 1991; 101(5):465–468.

32. Zhang F, Sprecher AJ, Wei C, Jiang JJ. Implantation of gelatin sponge combined with injection of autologous fat for sulcus vocalis. *Otolaryngol Head Neck Surg* 2010; 143(2):198–203.

33. Sataloff RT, Spiegel JR, Hawkshaw M, *et al.* Autologous fat implantation for vocal fold scar: a preliminary report *J Voice* 1997; 11(2):238–246.

34. Sataloff RT. Autologous fat implantation for vocal fold scar. *Curr Opin Otolaryngol Head Neck Surg* 2010; 18(6):503–506.

35. Tsunoda K, Takanosawa M, Niimi S. Autologous transplantation of fascia into the vocal fold: a new phonosurgical technique for glottal incompetence. *Laryngoscope* 1999; 109(3):504–508.

36. Wang CT, Liao LJ, Cheng PW, *et al.* Intralesional steroid injection for benign vocal fold disorders: a systematic review and meta-analysis. *Laryngoscope* 2013; 123(1):197–203.

37. Zhou H, Sivasankar M, Kraus DH, *et al.*Glucocorticoids regulate extracellular matrix metabolism in human vocal fold fibroblasts. *Laryngoscope* 2011; 121(9):1915–1919.

38. Hochman B, Locali RF, Matsuoka PK, Ferreira LM. Intralesional triamcinolone acetonide for keloid treatment: a systematic review. *Aesthet Surg J.* 2008; 32(4):705–709.

39. Mortensen M, Woo P. Office steroid injections of the larynx. *Laryngoscope* 2006; 116(10):1735–1739.

40. Mallur PS, Rosen CA. Vocal fold injection: review of indications, techniques, and materials for augmentation. *Clin Exp Otorhinolaryngol* 2010; 3(4):177–182.

41. Hsiung MW, Pai L. Autogenous fat injection for glottic insufficiency: analysis of 101 cases and correlation with patients' self-assessment. *Acta oto-laryngologica* 2006; 126(2):191–196.

42. Amin MR. Thyrohyoid approach for vocal fold augmentation. *Ann Otol Rhinol Laryngol* 2006; 115(9):699–702.

43. Ford CN, Martin DW, Warner TF. Injectable collagen in laryngeal rehabilitation. *Laryngoscope* 1984; 94(4):513–518.

44. Ford CN, Bless DM. Clinical experience with injectable collagen for vocal fold augmentation. *Laryngoscope* 1986; 96(8):863–869.

45. Molteni G, Bergamini G, Ricci-Maccarini A, *et al.* Auto-crosslinked hyaluronan gel injections in phonosurgery. *Otolaryngol Head Neck Surg* 2010; 142(4):547–553.

46. Kwon TK, Rosen CA, Gartner-Schmidt J. Preliminary results of a new temporary vocal fold injection material. *J Voice* 2005; 19(4):668–673.

47. Mallur PS, Morrison MP, Postma GN, *et al.* Safety and efficacy of carboxymethyl-cellulose in the treatment of glottic insufficiency. *Laryngoscope* 2012;122(2):322–326.

48. Moon IH, Park KN, Kim HK, Lee S. Utility and safety of commercially available injection laryngoplasty materials in a rabbit model. *J Voice* 2015; 29(1):125–128.

49. Carroll TL, Rosen CA. Long-term results of calcium hydroxylapatite for vocal fold augmentation. *Laryngoscope* 2011; 121(2):313–319.

50. DeFatta RA, Chowdhury FR, Sataloff RT. Complications of injection laryngo-plasty using calcium hydroxylapatite. *J Voice* 2012; 26(5):614–618.

51. Gray SD, Bielamowicz SA, Titze IR, *et al*. Experimental approaches to vocal fold alteration: introduction to the minithyrotomy. *Ann Otol Rhinol Laryngol* 1999; 108(1):1–9.

52. Mallur PS, Gartner-Schmidt J, Rosen CA. Voice outcomes following the gray minithyrotomy. *Ann Otol Rhinol Laryngol* 2012; 121(7):490–496.

53. Su CY, Tsai SS, Chiu JF, Cheng CA. Medialization laryngoplasty with strap muscle transposition for vocal fold atrophy with or without sulcus vocalis.. *Laryngoscope* 2004; 114(6):1106–1112.

54. Hirano S, Kishimoto Y, Suehiro A, *et al*. Regeneration of aged vocal fold: first human case treated with fibroblast growth factor. *Laryngoscope* Jan 2009; 119(1):197–202.

55. Hirano S, Mizuta M, Kaneko M, *et al*. Regenerative phonosurgical treatments for vocal fold scar and sulcus with basic fibroblast growth factor. *Laryngoscope* Nov 2013;123(11):2749–2755.

8

Laryngeal resurfacing

Joel E. Portnoy, Mary J. Hawkshaw, Robert T. Sataloff

Vocal fold injury, whether singular or repetitive, may damage the vocal folds' layered structure, interfering with inherent vibratory ability. Fortunately, most traumatic events of the vocal fold are repaired without incident, although several factors, including injury severity, an individual's healing capacity and local environmental factors, determine whether the effects of an injury endure. Trauma to the vocal fold mucosa and/or superficial lamina propria can result in stiffness that impairs mucosal mobility, leading to dysphonia. To date, no ideal replacement for the nascent superficial lamina propria exists, making vocal fold scar among the biggest challenges faced by caretakers of voice patients.

Although scar-like abnormalities can result from congenital malformations (e.g. sulcus vocalis), usually scar is the result of ongoing irritation and/or inflammation, direct mucosal trauma or phonotrauma, or laryngeal surgery. If the mucosal damage is severe, the mucosa tethers to underlying tissues obliterating vocal fold vibration. In these cases, epithelium-freeing procedures, and other techniques described elsewhere in this book are not always adequate to restore a straight, appropriately positioned mucosal surface, let alone a mucosal wave. Additionally, overresection of vocal fold mucosa can lead to loss of vocal fold bulk and glottic insufficiency, requiring replacement of the mucosa and underlying tissue. Such patients most commonly have experienced major laryngeal trauma or extensive cancer surgery, and large portions of the vocal fold require reconstruction to repair both glottic incompetence and non-vibrating mucosa. If a non-vibrating vocal fold is scarred laterally so far that glottic closure is impossible, and when the involved vocal fold is scarred so densely that mucosa can not be separated and reconfigured to allow fat implantation, or when the scar involves the hemilarynx so densely that the vocal fold can not be medialized adequately even with thyroplasty, vocal fold resurfacing is appropriate.

Scar resection (Figures 1A-I)

Whether approached endoscopically or open, complete resection of the scarred mucosal surface is vital to proper reconstruction. (Figures 8.1A-I) After palpation of the scar to assess extent and severity, hydrodissection is performed via subepithelial infusion with 1% lidocaine with 1:100,000 epinephrine. In severe scar, this does not elevate the mucosa, but it provides vasoconstriction, After vasoconstriction occurs, a straight Sataloff sharp knife is utilized to incise the mucosa on the superior surface of the vocal fold about a millimeter lateral to the residual medial edge. Straight microscissors are used to dissect the scar from the underlying vocal ligament, (if present) or muscle, on the depth of the scar. Incisions are made with the straight microscissors delineating the anterior and posterior extent of the resection. A curved spatula is utilized to define the deep extent of the dissection bluntly when possible. Following complete elevation, the scar to be excised is grasped and stabilized with a heart-shaped forceps and resected using curved microscissors. It is critical to remove the medial mucosa and scar entirely so that no stiff mucosa or tissue is inadvertently buried with the resurfacing graft. If the scar extends deeply into the muscle, partial resection to avoid creating an excessive defect may be considered. The resultant defect determines how reconstruction proceeds.

Reconstruction

Free tissue grafting and local flaps are two reconstructive options utilized to resurface areas of tissue loss. In otolaryngology, free tissue grafts are used in various procedures such as tympanoplasty, rhinoplasty and laryngotracheal reconstruction. These grafts rely on the recipient site tissues for blood supply and carry risk of failure due to avascular necrosis. Resurfacing of laryngeal wounds is important to avoid infection, granulation tissue, and in the case of vocal fold mucosa, dysphonia from severe scarring. Several tissues have been suggested for resurfacing of the laryngeal tissues, but mucosal grafting typically provides the best results.[1,2,3]

Figure 8.1A-I: Vocal Fold Scar Resection (from Surgical Techniques in Otolaryngology – Head and Neck Surgery, Laryngeal Surgery, Page 121, pictures A-I). Images reproduced by permission of Jaypee Brothers Medical Publishers

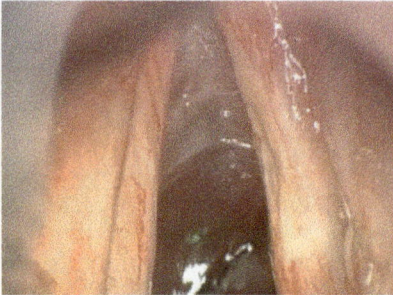

A: Nonvibrating, depressed scar along the right musculomembranous vocal fold.

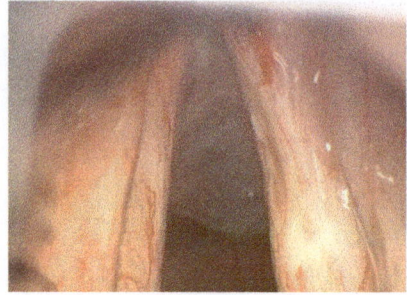

B: Subepithelial infusion with 1% lidocaine and 1:100,000 epinephrine distends the superficial lamina propria and vasoconstricts its microvasculature.

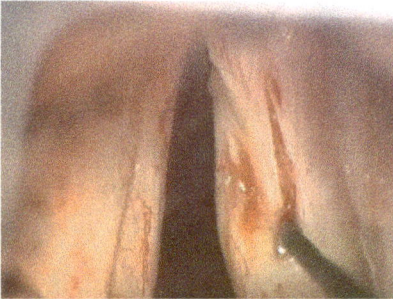

C: An incision is made at the superolateral extent of the scar.

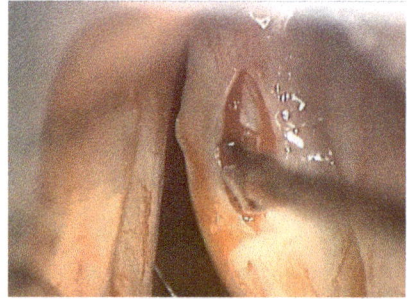

D: Straight microscissors are used to create a minimicroflap.

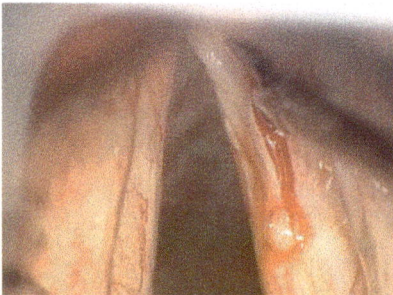

E: Straight microscissors are used to make the anterior cut.

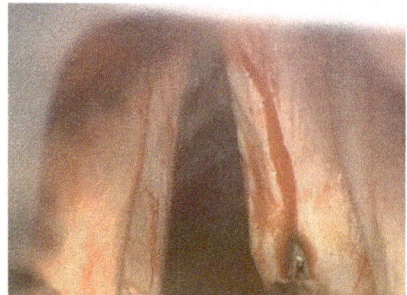

F: Straight microscissors are also used to make the posterior cut.

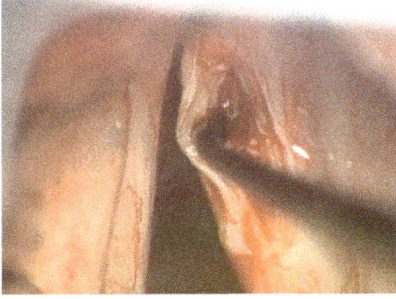

G: Blunt dissection is performed with a curved spatula separating scar from the underlying vocal ligament.

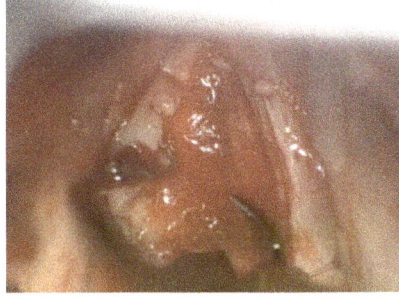

H: The scar is stabilized with heart-shaped forceps and resected with microscissors.

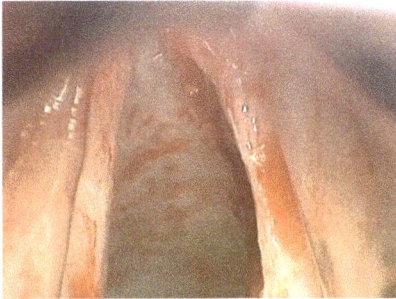

I: The resulting defect involves nearly the entire length of the right musculomembranous vocal fold.

Buccal mucosa, as suggested by Isshiki[4], has been established as a reasonable donor tissue due to its ease of harvest, lack of donor morbidity, variable thickness and ability to contain underlying fat to support some vocal fold vibration. The buccal graft should be about 20% larger than the vocal fold defect to allow for contracture.

External approaches

In the most extreme cases, it might be necessary to resect the scarred vocal fold and create a pseudo vocal fold using strap muscle flaps, a technique employed commonly following cordectomy or hemilaryngectomy[5,6]. This procedure is performed through an external approach. The thyroid cartilage is opened by laryngofissure, and a small portion of cartilage is removed at the level of the vocal fold, lateral to the midline. The surgical steps are as follows:

An incision is planned in a horizontal neck crease approximately half way along the middle over the thyroid lamina. The skin and subcutaneous tissues are infused with 1% lidocaine with 1:100,000 epinephrine. After waiting for vasoconstriction to occur, an incision is made through the skin and platysma. Small subplatysmal flaps are developed. The strap muscles are divided in the midline and retracted laterally, providing exposure of the thyroid ala.

The thyroid lamina is separated vertically approximately 5mm lateral to the midline in a paramedian position on the ipsilateral side of the reconstruction using a #15 scalpel or oscillating saw. When necessary because of anterior vocal fold deficiency, the cartilage incision can be closer to the midline. Violation of the laryngeal introitus and resection of inner perichondrium are avoided. The inner perichondrium is elevated delicately from the inner surface of the thyroid cartilage. The thyrohyoid and cricothyroid membranes are incised until the ipsilateral thyroid lamina can be retracted laterally.

The bipedicled strap muscle flap usually consists of the sternoyhoid muscle, although the sternothyroid, omohyoid and/or thyrohyoid muscles can be incorporated as needed to create more bulk, if necessary. Some surgeons have recommended using ipsilateral strap muscle. However, the senior author (RTS) prefers rotating contralateral strap muscle because it can be positioned directly to replace the true vocal fold muscle without having to be bent, as it would if it were coming from the same side. The strap muscle can be left uncovered to heal by secondary intention, or it can be covered with buccal mucosa or mucosa harvested from within the larynx. The authors prefer harvest of supraglottic laryngeal mucosa, if the patient has not been radiated and the mucosa is not involved in scar, and if the patient is not dependant on false vocal fold phonation. The muscle flap is mobilized along its lateral border without violating the cephalic or caudal attachments containing its blood supply. Sometimes, the caudal edge of the thyroid lamina can be trimmed slightly with a small burr to allow for a smooth transition into the larynx (preventing pinching of the vascular supply). The muscle is then transposed into the space between the thyroid lamina and the paraglottic soft tissues. The thyroid cartilage is then re-approximated using with 2-0 Prolene® or 0.4 to 0.45 mm stainless wires. Hemostasis is achieved and the wound is closed in multiple layers with absorbable sutures.

Reconstruction can also be performed through a midline laryngofissure, removing a small ipsilateral cartilage window, and transposing a monopedicle muscle flap with or without mucosal covering.

Other resurfacing techniques can be performed through a laryngofissure, including buccal graft, vocal fold flap, false vocal fold graft or flap and others. These operations are technically easier to perform through a laryngofissure, but they also can be performed endoscopically. The endoscopic approach is preferred by the authors, as described in the next section, unless muscle is needed to reconstruct the body of the vocal fold.

Lateral external approaches

It is not necessary to perform a laryngofissure to achieve the goals of the procedure discussed above. Although exposure for suturing is somewhat limited, the vocal fold can be resurfaced and grafted from a lateral approach, especially when vocal fold scar and lateralization are so severe that the vocal fold is virtually absent. In such cases, a lateral thyrotomy is performed in a matter similar to a classic thyroplasty. A window roughly 6 x 10-1 2 mm is opened. If more exposure is needed superiorly or inferiorly, additional cartilage can be resected; but extending the thyrotomy too far superiorly is a disadvantage to accurate placement of a thyroplasty, should thyroplasty be required at a future stage. Through the lateral approach, the scarred tissue and mucosa can be resected, buccal graft can be sutured to replace the surface (from inside out), and a strap muscle can be rotated to fill the defect. When possible, the strap muscle rotation flap should be based superiorly. This minimizes tension on the muscle flap when the larynx rises during the swallowing. The interior aspect of the muscle is divided, making the rotation flap long enough to avoid any tension on the muscle when the larynx is raised or lowered. The inferior aspect of the muscle is rotated into the larynx through the thyrotomy, and is used to reconstitute the bulk of the body of the vocal fold. Approximately 20% over correction is desirable. The sides of the muscle flap are sutured to the thyroid cartilage at the edges of the thyrotomy. This helps stabilize the flap within the larynx and helps prevent displacement of the flap during laryngeal or neck movement.

Endoscopic approaches

Endoscopic approaches frequently reduce perioperative morbidity. Teamed with advances in the endoscopic instrumentation, minimally invasive techniques are being developed that achieve results previously feasible only by external approaches.

Buccal graft harvesting and placement (Figures 2A-F)

Free tissue grafting is performed typically in a single procedure. The buccal harvest site is prepared by infiltrating 1% lidocaine with 1:100,000 epinephrine. An incision through the mucosa is made using a #15 scalpel and is carried into the underlying fat. A composite graft containing both mucosa and buccal fat is harvested, and the donor site is closed with absorbable sutures. The graft is then inserted into the laryngoscope and oriented with the fat facing the freshly incised vocal fold. Fibrin glue may be placed between the graft and recipient site. The graft is sutured in place, starting with the inferior aspect, followed by placement additional sutures to ensure the graft is stable enough to resist being dislodged by a cough. The sutures are cut. Graft stability is critical as mobility of the graft can lead to poor healing or graft failure. The patient is extubated deeply with the laryngoscope in place to trauma to the graft.

False vocal fold flap harvest and placement (Figures 3A-3T)

It is not always necessary to harvest graft material from a distant site (e.g. buccal mucosa). Free tissue grafts can be harvested from the false vocal fold. Supraglottic tissue also can be rotated as a vascularized flap. Similar to free tissue grafts, local flaps, such as the paramedian forehead flap and the pectoralis major myocutaneous flap are used widely in reconstruction of head and neck defects. Many of these flaps offer not only epithelial tissue, but also subepithelial bulk, allowing for reconstruction of vital deep tissues. These flaps rely on the established donor site blood supply while the flap vasculature invests into the local tissues. Because these flaps do not rely on the surrounding tissues for their vascular supply, they can be inset into more poorly vascularized areas, such as over cartilage or in irradiated fields. False vocal fold rotation flaps follow these principles and work well.

Figure 8.2A-F: Buccal Mucosal Graft Reconstruction (from Surgical Techniques in Otolaryngology – Head and Neck Surgery, Laryngeal Surgery, Page 121, pictures J-O). Images reproduced by permission of Jaypee Medical Publishers

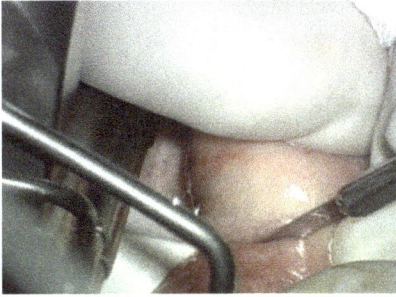

A: A buccal incision is made with a scalpel through the mucosa and carried into the submucosal fat.

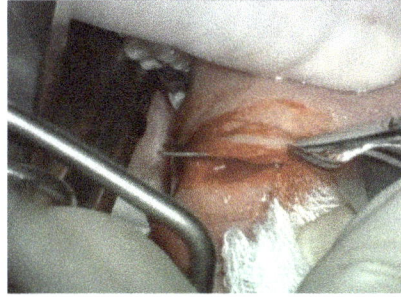

B: A composite graft containing fat is harvested; the fat will act as filler replacing the absent superficial lamina propria allowing the overlying buccal mucosa to vibrate.

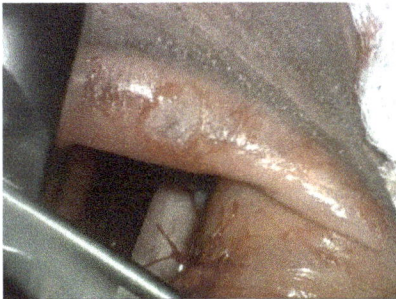

C: The buccal incision is closed with 3-0 chromic sutures.

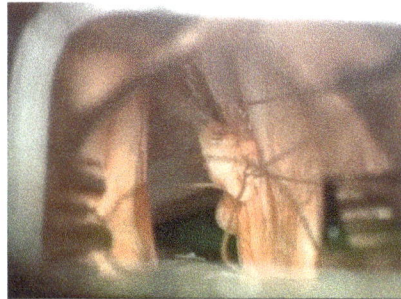

D: The buccal mucosal graft is placed into position ensuring proper orientation. Size and positioning can be adjusted until optimal configuration is achieved.

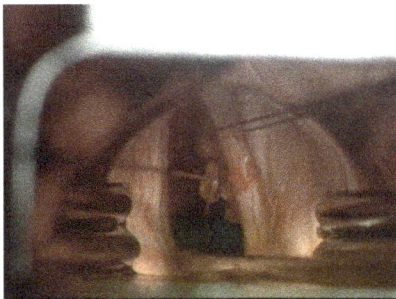

E: Multiple sutures secure the graft in position and the excess suture is trimmed.

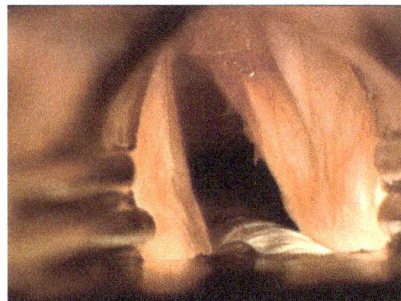

F: The graft is in position. A deep extubation is performed and the patient is kept on strict voice rest until seen for outpatient follow-up examination in 7 days.

Figure 8.3A-T: False Vocal Fold Flap Reconstruction

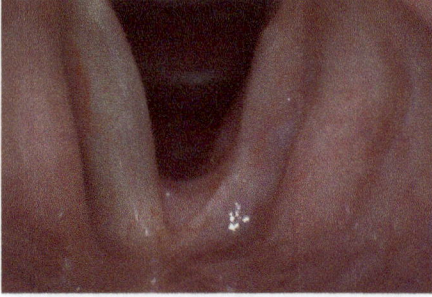

A: Preoperative strobovideolaryngoscopy revealing a scarred defect on abduction of a patient who has undergone resection of glottic carcinoma, adjuvant radiotherapy and has failed voice therapy and lipoimplantation. A pedicled flap is favored due to the presumed poor vascular supply in the area (radiation, surgery).

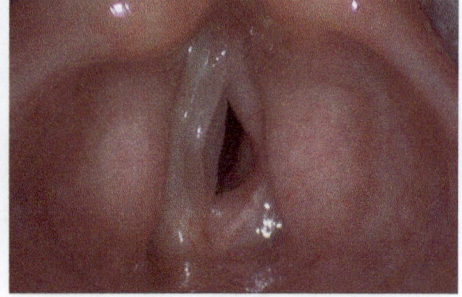

B: Preoperative strobovideolaryngoscopy showing glottic insufficiency during phonation.

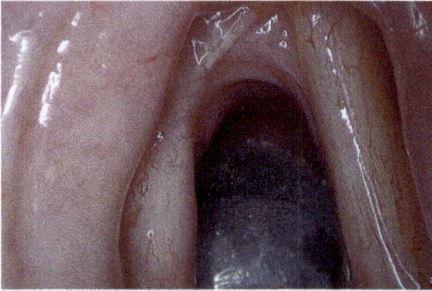

C: Operative view via a 0-degree telescope of defect preoperatively revealing a thick, scarred keyhole deformity.

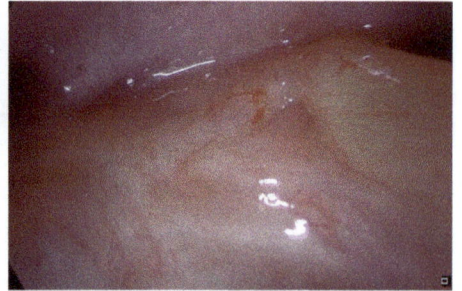

D: 70-degree telescope view of the defect preoperatively, showing a lack of 3 layers of the vocal fold anteriorly.

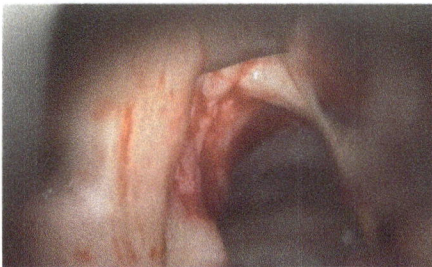

E: Existing scar at the recipient site is resected.

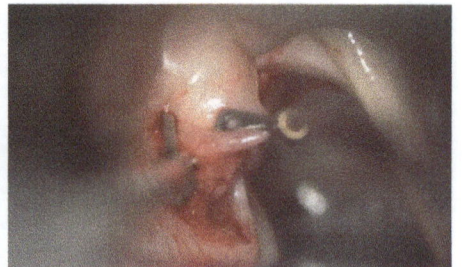

F: The false vocal fold is injected with lidocaine with epinephrine and transected at the posterior margin laterally. Next, dissection occurs at the lateral margin in an anterior direction.

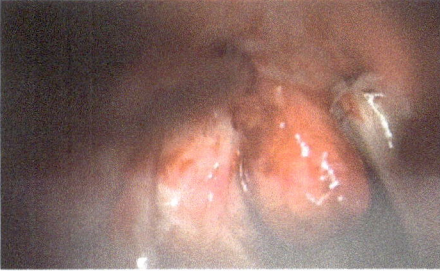

G: The false vocal fold flap has been created and is noticeably smaller now that it is no longer under tension.

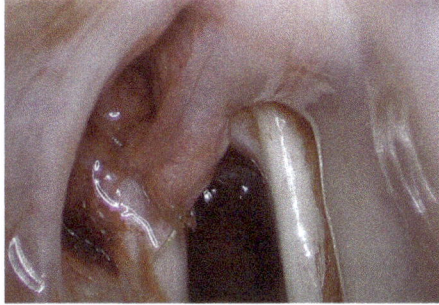

H: The false vocal fold is secured, inferiorly first, using chromic sutures tied endoscopically and the tails are trimmed.

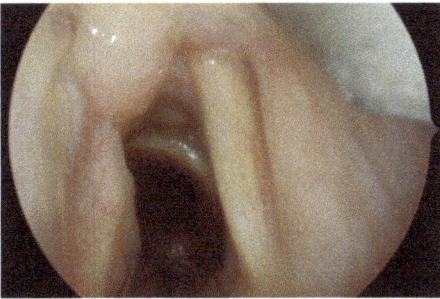

I: 3 weeks later, the patient returns to the operating theater for takedown of the flap. On this 0-degree telescopic view, it is apparent that the flap has retracted superiorly, accounting for the patient's suboptimal voice after the first procedure.

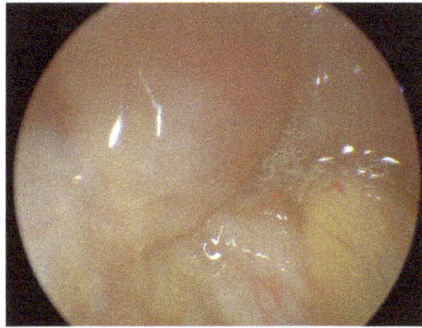

J: Preoperative 70-degree telescopic view reveals that the false vocal fold flap has taken to the recipient site, but is at a slight height mismatch from the right vocal fold (yellow, seen at the right).

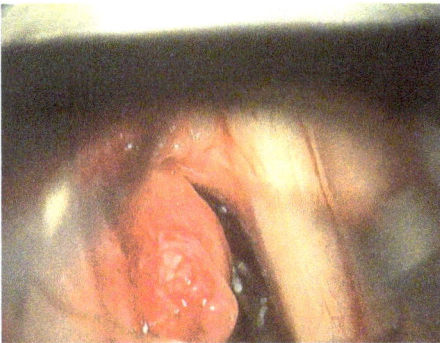

K: First, the anterior pedicle of the flap is transected, ensuring that the deep or lateral aspect of the flap remains attached to its new blood supply.

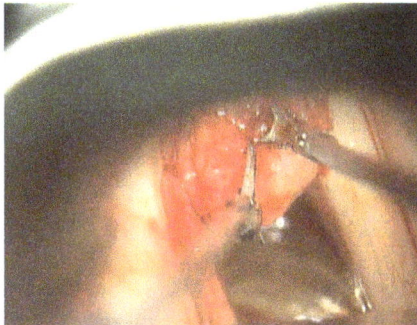

L: It is possible to debulk some of the false vocal fold flap if excess is though to be present. Caution should be taken no to over-resect submucosal tissue, as it is likely to retract and atrophy somewhat before the final result is seen.

127

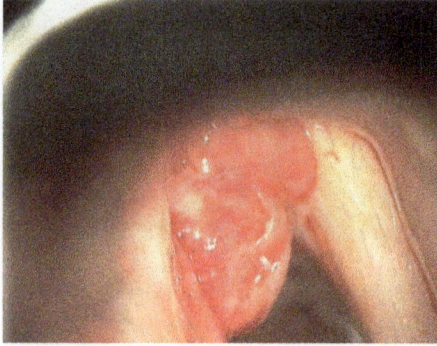

M: The false vocal fold flap is inset into position.

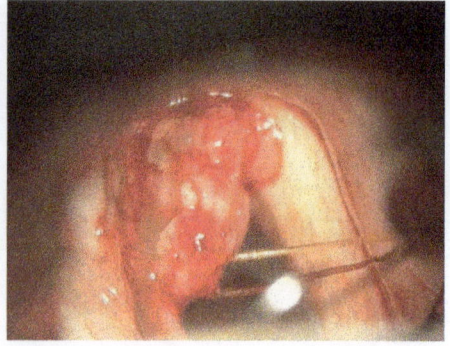

N: The flap is secured into place with chromic sutures tied endoscopically. The suture tails are trimmed. The flap edges can be secured further with tissue sealant.

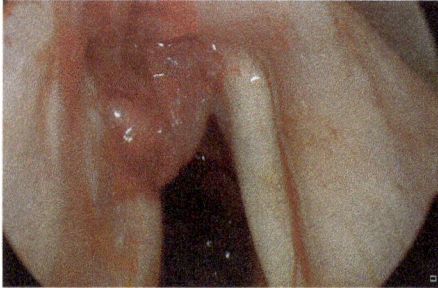

O: Final operative view via 0-degree telescope.

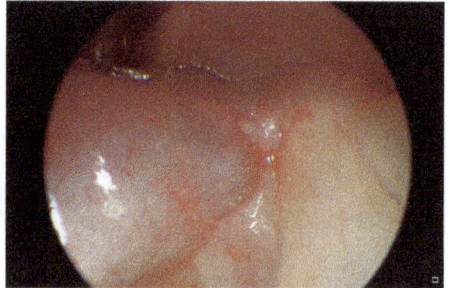

P: Final operative view via 70-degree telescope.

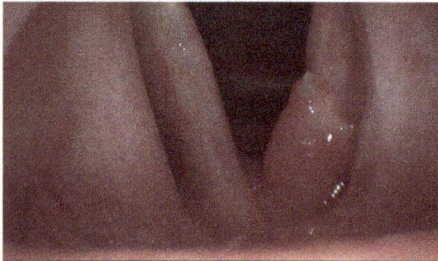

Q: 1 month later, the patient noted substantially improved projection, reduced vocal fatigue and enhanced clarity. Strobovideolaryngoscopy revealed continued healing of the flap.

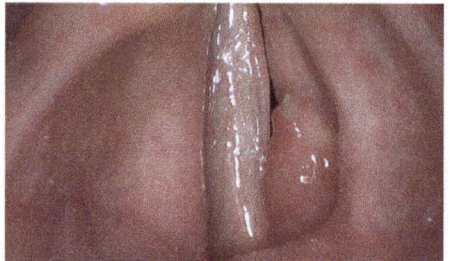

R: Phonation revealed much improved glottic closure on strobovideolaryngoscopy.

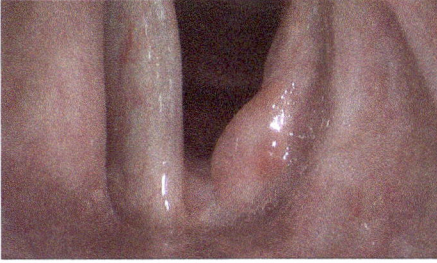

S: 3 months postoperatively, the patient still reported improved vocal outcome with further thinning of the flap.

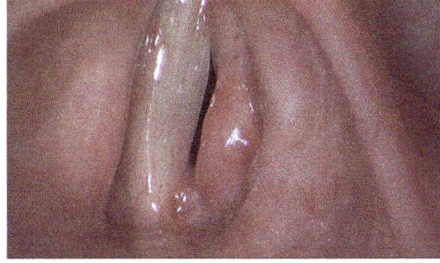

T: During phonation, vibration is seen throughout the false vocal fold flap, though a small amount of glottic insufficiency has developed.

In hemilaryngectomy and large defects, pedicled strap muscle flaps, such as the sternohyoid flap, can be utilized for reconstruction of large defects as discussed above. Similarly, the false vocal fold, or ventricular fold, can be harvested to reconstruct the vocal fold using open approaches[7,8], but also can be performed in a purely endoscopic approach, as described below. The ventricular fold is supplied by branches of the superior and inferior thyroid arteries. These branches can be encountered during vocal cordotomy, performed for neoplastic or airway indications. Due to the lack of a large, named vessel supplying this area, the false vocal fold flap can be pedicled either anteriorly or posteriorly, depending on the defect requiring reconstruction. It has the advantage of likely improved survival in a field with challenged vascularity such as following radiation, or severe trauma and scar.

If the patient has full, healthy false vocal folds, and if he/she is not using the false vocal folds as the phonatory source of oscillation (compensatory ventricular phonation), then the false vocal fold tissue can make an excellent material for resurfacing the true vocal fold. False vocal fold flap reconstruction is performed in a staged fashion, although some cases do not require the second procedure should the patient and surgeon be satisfied with the outcome. In a first procedure, the defect, or recipient site, is prepared as described above (scar resection). If the defect was created freshly, the edges should be straightened as much as possible to accommodate a relatively straight flap. If the donor site has healed, the area should be de-epithelialized allowing for fresh, healing tissue to be at the intersection of the donor and recipient sites.

Once the vocal fold is prepared, replacement tissue is harvested from the false vocal fold. Like a buccal graft, the false vocal graft should be at 20% larger than necessary, to account for contraction during healing. If it remains too large, it can be trimmed at a later date. To harvest a false vocal fold graft, a through-and-through incision is made, and the desired portion of the false vocal fold is repositioned inferiorly to replace the medial portion of the true vocal fold. It is stabilized with fibrin glue and sutures and is effective in replacing much of the multilayered structure of the vocal fold following tissue loss. Like the buccal graft, a free false vocal fold graft can be dislodged and lost, by forceful coughing, for example; Three to four weeks after the initial procedure, a second procedure can be performed to divide the pedicle, trim the flap and further rotate it for optimal positioning.

In order to create a false vocal fold flap, incisions are made in the false vocal fold only anteriorly or posteriorly. The choice of an anteriorly based or posteriorly based flap is determined by the position of the area that needs to be replaced on the true vocal fold, and by the size and shape of the false vocal fold. The end to be rotated should be as broad as possible, as should the base (to retain blood supply). The false vocal fold flap is rotated inferiorly and sutured to the inferior border of the vocal fold defect. The rotation flap usually is divided during a separate microlaryngoscopic procedure approximately six weeks later. At that time, the flap is integrated well inferiorly. The flap can be divided, shaped, and the superior vocal fold mucosal reconstruction can be sutured to complete the procedure. The remnant of the flap can be repositioned in the false vocal fold, or discarded. When possible, the authors prefer to reposition it both to preserve potentially useful tissue for future procedures, and to preserve false vocal fold aerodynamic vocal fold function (down-stream resistance). In addition to the advantage of being vascularized, the false vocal fold flap also has the advantage of remaining attached to the body. Although coughing off buccal grafts or false fold free grafts is not common, it can occur. If a cough injures a false vocal fold rotation flap, the flap is not lost; it is necessary only to resuture the flap to salvage the procedure.

Postoperative care

Resurfacing procedures using grafts and flaps are delicate. Voice rest is required for at least one week. Patients are examined at that time to determine whether gentle phonation appears safe, based on the stability of the graft. Antitussive medications (such as benzonatate pearls) are begun preoperatively and continued postoperatively. Straining should also be avoided, in some cases necessitating usage of laxatives. When voice rest is discontinued, a speech language pathologist, ideally a therapist with whom the patient had worked prior to surgery, facilitates the patient's transition to modified voice rest.

It is often necessary to adjust and reshape the graft. In general, we recommended waiting a minimum of six months, unless there is such excessive graft tissue (usually far anteriorly) that unacceptable trauma is being cause to the contralateral vocal fold. The most common adjustment required is debulking the graft or flap anteriorly. This should be done submucosally through an incision on the superior surface, except when it is also necessary to resect some of the surface tissue. If the replaced surface is not sufficiently pliable, submucosal fat implantation (as described in the chapter on epithelium freeing techniques) can be performed. While it is probably safe after six months, the senior author (RTS) recommends waiting one year, when possible. This not only assures that the free graft or flap has healed fully, but it also allows sufficient time for spontaneous return of mucosal wave and softening of the medial surface (which sometimes take a year, or even slightly longer). In some cases, the need for fat implantation can be avoided by transferring fat at the first stage. Buccal fat can be left attached to the mucosal graft, and platysmal fat can be harvested and placed between a mucosal graft and strap muscle through a thyrotomy; fat can be harvested from the neck or abdomen and placed through a lateral approach between the sutured mucosal graft and the rotated strap muscle flap. It is reasonable to place fat at the time of the initial procedure. If it extrudes or even scars, little is lost. If it remains soft, chances of a good result without additional surgery are increased.

Conclusion

In this age of rapid medical advancement, successful transplantation of a growing number of organs and tissue engineering hold promise for laryngeal reconstruction. Although scaffolding and tissue engineering have shown promise for reconstruction of large defects of the larynx[9], the successful reconstruction of the complex, multi-layered vocal fold with its specialized mucosa and superficial lamina propria continues to elude medical science. Ongoing research is seeking the so-called 'holy grail' of vocal fold reconstruction (re-engineered, layered vocal fold); but for now, reasonable voice outcomes can be obtained with free mucosal grafting and local flaps. The vast majority of patients with vocal fold scar can be improved through more conservative measures. However, techniques are available to help even those with profound vocal fold scar, or absence of a vocal fold. Results usually are gratifying, but almost never perfect; and staged procedures are routine. It is essential for patients to understand the likely multi-staged course, and to have reasonable expectations regarding outcomes. When performed correctly, these procedures have little donor site morbidity, and substantial improvement in phonatory quality and effort.

References

1. Hirano M, Kurita S, Matsuoka H. Vocal function following hemilaryngectomy. *Ann Otol Rhinol Laryngol* 1987; 96(5):586–589.
2. Isshiki N, Taira T, Nose K, Kojima H. Surgical treatment of laryngeal web with mucosa graft. *Ann Otol Rhinol Laryngol* 1991; 100(2):95–100.
3. Andrews RJ, Blackwell KE, Berke GS, *et al.* Combined buccal mucosa island and sternohyoid flaps: a new technique of hemilaryngeal reconstruction studied in a canine model. *Ann Otol Rhinol Laryngol* 2001; 110(6):543–549.
4. Isshiki N. Recent advances in phonosurgery. *Folia Phoniatr* 1980; 32(2):119–154.
5. Spiegel JR, Sataloff RT. Surgery for carcinoma of the larynx. In: Gould WJ, Sataloff RT, Spiegel JR (Eds). *Voice Surgery.* St. Louis, MO: CV Mosby Co 1993; 307–338
6. Bailey BJ. Glottic reconstruction after hemilaryngectomy: bipedicle muscle flap laryngoplasty. *Laryngoscope* 1975; 85(6): 960–977.
7. Brasnu D, Laccourreye O, Weinstein G, *et al.* False vocal cord reconstruction of the glottis following vertical partial laryngectomy: a preliminary analysis *Laryngoscope* 1992; 102:717–719.
8. Biacabe B, Crevier-Buchman L, Hans S, *et al.* Phonatory mechanisms after vertical partial laryngectomy with glottic reconstruction by false vocal fold flap. *Ann Otol Rhinol Laryngol* 2001; 110(10):935–940.
9. Kitani Y, Kanemaru S, Umeda H, *et al.* Laryngeal regeneration using tissue engineering techniques in a canine model. *Ann Otol Rhinol Laryngol* 2011; 120(1):49–56.

9

Lasers

Inna Husain and Ramon A. Franco Jr.

Introduction

Since their first use in otolaryngology in the 1960s, lasers have quickly become an integral part of the surgical armamentarium for the laryngologist. The development of the micromanipulator[1] that allowed the delivery of the carbon dioxide (CO_2) laser beam coupled to a microscope is considered the beginning of modern laryngeal laser surgery. Further advancements led to the use of laser technology via flexible endoscopes allowing routine use in the outpatient setting as well. Although laser use in laryngeal microsurgery is well established, one emerging area of use is in the treatment of vocal fold scars. In order to select the best laser for the respective pathology in the larynx, the surgeon must have a good understanding of basic laser physiology and tissue interactions.

Carbon dioxide laser

The first laser to be used in otolaryngology and considered to be the workhorse in laryngology is the CO_2 laser. Its specific wavelength of 10,600nm is selectively absorbed by water found in soft tissues. It can emit continuous waves which can be focused into a thin beam for incision, excision or to vaporize and ablate tissue. Ideal indications for use include glottic, subglottic, or tracheal stenosis resections, arytenoidectomy or transverse cordotomy for airway compromise from stenosis that can result from vocal fold paralysis, or resection of early-stage glottic squamous cell carcinomas. It also has good hemostatic capabilities when addressing blood vessels less than 0.5mm in diameter. Although for selective lesions the CO_2 laser's advantages of hemostasis, improved visibility, and less tissue manipulation are compelling, heat-induced consequences should not be overlooked. Lateral thermal energy spread has been reported to delay healing and increase scar formation. The most significant disadvantage to the use of the CO_2 laser in laryngeal surgery is thermal injury to the intermediate and deep layers of the lamina propria. With this increased risk of injury to the lamina propria, the use of the CO_2 laser for benign masses of the vocal fold, including sulcus deformities and scar, is the subject of much debate as it may induce more scarring post-operatively[2].

Angiolytic lasers

Angiolytic lasers operate on the principle of selective photothermolysis as described first by Anderson and Parrish. In this principle, each laser beam is absorbed by a specific chromophore target and damages that chromophore by conversion into thermal energy and minimizing thermal damage to surrounding tissue. Optimal characteristics of the laser to ensure thermolysis include a wavelength absorbed by the target chromophore, an action time shorter than the thermal relaxation time of the target (amount of time to dissipate the heat), and enough fluence (laser energy over the surface area treated in J/cm^2) to reach a sufficient temperature to destroy the chromophore[3]. Therefore, the variables for the clinician to select while working with photoangiolytic lasers include the wavelength, the pulse duration, energy setting, spot size, and distance to the target tissue.

In recent years, there has been a shift from the use of the CO_2 laser in laryngology to the use of the 532nm potassium titanyl phosphate (KTP) laser and the 585nm pulsed dye laser (PDL) (Figures 9.1 and 9.2). These lasers are classified as angiolytic, due to their vascular selectivity with wavelengths that closely correspond to oxyhemoglobin absorption peaks of 542 and 577 nm respectively. Both lasers have a penetration depth of 1–2mm and are delivered via a thin (0.6–0.2mm) glass fiber, allowing for use through a flexible laryngoscope side channel making office-based laser procedures possible. The KTP laser has a slightly lower bleeding rate when compared to the PDL laser. This higher rate in the PDL laser has been attributed to the short pulse duration which delivers energy in a shorter time, rapidly heating the microvasculature resulting in potential vessel rupture. This is a shortcoming of the version of the PDL used in otolaryngology, which lacks the ability to change the pulse duration. The KTP laser, however, is adjustable and, when set to a longer pulse duration, results in a lower potential for vessel rupture. By using the 'pulse stacking technique', the risk of vessel rupture can be reduced when using the PDL laser. This involves starting the laser use at a further distance (1cm) and moving closer to the target as one progresses[4-6].

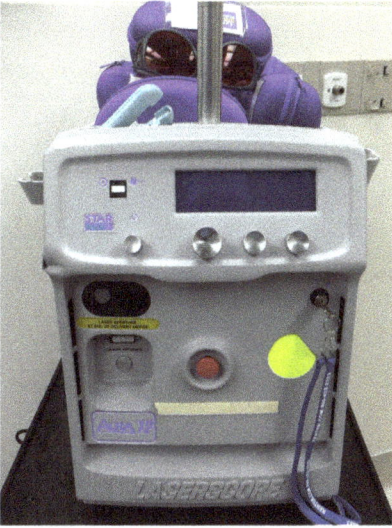

Figure 9.1. The 532nm- potassium titanyl phosphate (KTP) laser with the ability to adjust pulse duration. Orange colored protective glasses are provided to all persons in the treatment room. Photo courtesy of Inna Husain.

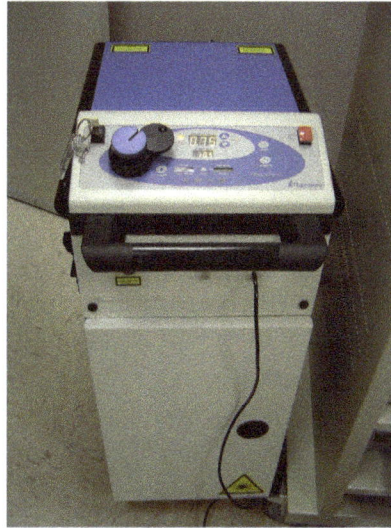

Figure 9.2. The 585nm pulsed dye laser (PDL). Purple-Blue colored protective glasses are worn. Photo courtesy of Inna Husain.

The pulsed-KTP laser is routinely used in the treatment of vascular lesions, papillomatosis, and dysplasia; while the PDL laser has been used in a variety of applications in laryngology over the past decade, including surgical management of papillomatosis, vascular polyps, leukoplakia, granulomas, and Reinke's edema. The PDL was first used in the dermatologic treatment of port-wine stains and telangiectasias. Work in the dermatologic literature has highlighted the effectiveness of the PDL for the treatment of fresh and well-established hypertrophic and keloid scars as well as scarring resulting from acne excoriee[7,8]. Even though the CO_2 laser can produce more dramatic skin resurfacing effects via its ablative properties, significant side effects including risk of permanent hyperpigmentation, delayed re-epithelialization, and prolonged erythema exist. Since the PDL demonstrates positive outcomes without major side effects, it has become the laser of choice for treatment of cutaneous scars[8].

Pulse dye laser

The biological mechanism of PDL-induced tissue change in the vocal fold and improved vocal fold scar has been explored on both a histological and transcriptional level. The mechanisms of action by which the PDL affects scarring have been proposed. They include heat-induced vasculitis leading to ischemia and nutrient deprivation to the scar, interference in collagen deposition, decreased expression of transforming growth factor beta-1 (TGF-B1), and an increase in the number of mast cells demonstrating potential ways that scar can be modulated at various stages of wound healing[5,9,10]. By targeting blood vessels, the PDL may essentially starve the treated area from receiving pro-inflammatory cytokines thereby decreasing the inflammation time. Also, PDL-treated samples have shown a coarsening of collagen fibers within the superficial lamina propria (Figure 9.3).This may suggest a target for collagenase and remodeling of scar[11].

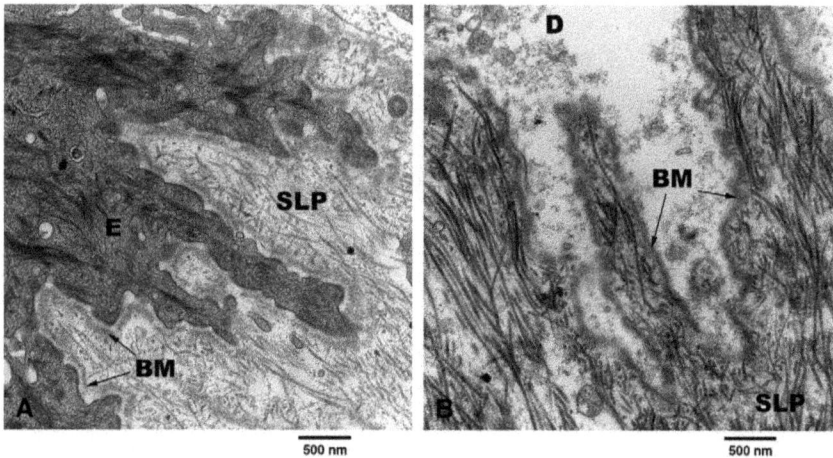

Figure 9.3 A. (electron microscopy 25,000x) High magnification view of the normal relationship of epithelial cells (E) to the basement membrane (BM) and superficial lamina propria (SLP). Fine collagen bundles can be observed within the SLP. B. (electron microscopy 25,000x) PDL treated samples demonstrate loss of basal epithelial cells due to separation of the epithelium from the basement membrane. Note the close relationship between the basement membrane and the SLP as the area previously occupied by basal epithelial cells is replaced by cellular debris (D). The collagen bundles are now coarse within the SLP[12].

Ayala *et al* examined vocal fold tissue samples from PDL-treated vocal folds with light microscopy, as well as transmission electron microscopy. When compared to control samples, the PDL-treated samples demonstrated a preferentially destroyed intraepithelial desmosome junction and coagulation of regional blood vessels. This consistently allowed for a separation of epithelial cells away from the basement membrane[11] (Figure 9.4). This suggests that the PDL beam passes unabsorbed through the epithelial layer and exerts its thermal effect on the lamina propria, confirming selective photothermolysis (Figure 9.4). Histologic analysis of normal rat vocal folds after PDL irradiation does show initial lamina propria edema and red blood cell infiltrate that, over time, converts to a neutrophilic infiltrate with vascular thrombosis and by one month, returns to normal morphology. Therefore, an inflammatory repair process was initiated in vivo after PDL irradiation and was completed by one month, with preservation of normal tissue morphology. Molecular analysis of rat vocal folds in vivo, and vocal fold fibroblasts in vitro after PDL irradiation, demonstrated altered inflammatory cytokine and procollagen/collagenase expression at the transcript level, parallel that which is seen in the dermatologic literature, supporting the theory that the PDL increases turnover of the extracellular matrix of the vocal fold. Therefore, the microscopic changes that happen in the lamina propria with scarring, for example an increase in type I and type III collagen, could be altered by the PDL, resulting in improved mucosal pliability and, thus, improved vocal fold vibration and voice[10]. While this work demonstrated that the PDL has the potential to modulate extracellular matrix (ECM) turnover, future studies should examine these changes in a disordered ECM model as seen in scar.

Due to the histopathology similarities between sulcus vocalis and scar tissue, as well as the prior use of PDL for other benign laryngeal lesions, the PDL was suggested as a new treatment modality for vocal fold scars[13]. Mortensen *et al* published the first reported use in their prospective study of 11 subjects with vocal fold scar treated with three serial in-office treatments with PDL. Subjects were followed for six months post-treatment and there was a significant improvement in the total Voice Handicap Index (VHI) score, as well as every subcategory. Additionally, there was improvement of acoustical voice parameters including jitter, shimmer, and noise-to-harmonic ratio. Blinded pre- and post-treatment videostroboscopic examinations demonstrated better vibration, mucosal wave amplitude, and decreased hyperemia. This study suggests that the key to achieving success in the treatment of vocal fold scar may be the return of vocal fold pliability[13]. Similarly, Hwang *et al* demonstrated statistically significant improvements in post-operative voice indices including VHI data, auditory perceptual judgment, and several of the acoustic and aerodynamic evaluation methods in their series of 25 patients undergoing PDL glottoplasty for sulcus vocalis[9].

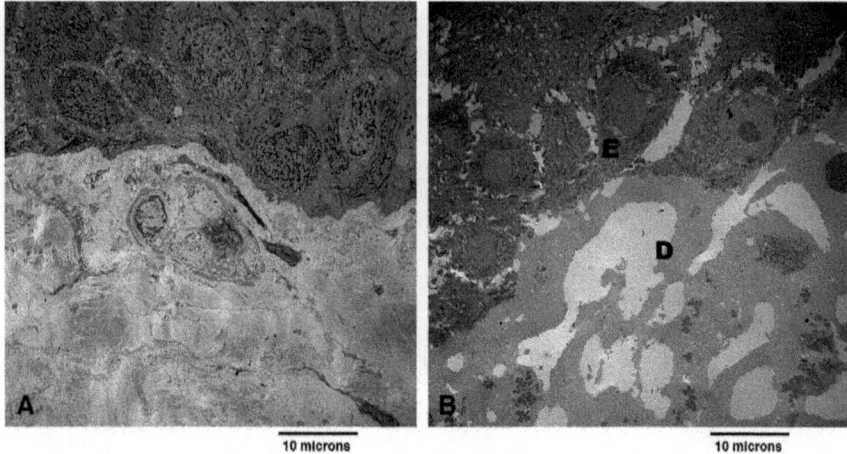

Figure 9.4. A. (electron microscopy 1900x) Normal appearance of the epithelial-superficial lamina propria junction. Note the intimate contact of the epithelial cells to the basement membrane. B. (electron microscopy 1900x) After treatment with the PDL, there is consistent separation of the epithelial cells (E) away from the basement membrane. Areas where the basement membrane-superficial lamina propria would normally be are replaced by cellular debris (D)[12].

KTP Laser

While the PDL has shown promise in the treatment of vocal fold scar, the use of the KTP laser in modulating vocal fold scar has not been clearly demonstrated in the literature. Sheu *et al* recently published a report in which vocal folds in a rat model were subjected to injury and underwent therapeutic treatment with the KTP. Although an additive effect on inflammatory gene expression and matrix metalloproteinase gene expression were seen temporarily, there was little impact on vocal fold fibrosis on histological analysis[14]. This lack of histologic modulation suggests that a single treatment of therapeutic KTP may not be sufficient to modulate vocal fold scar and repeated treatments, as performed by Mortensen *et al*[9] with the PDL, may be necessary. In addition, the temporary and limited upregulation of extracellular matrix (ECM) metabolism mediators proposes a role for multiple modality treatment for vocal fold scar. Therapy with an angiolytic laser treatment along with adjuvant treatment with, for example, corticosteroids or 5-fluorouracil, may improve outcomes as seen in treatment for cutaneous scars[15].

Photoangiolytic lasers show promise in the treatment and modulation of vocal fold scar and suggest the ability to improve vocal fold stiffness and thereby improve voice outcomes. Clinical, histologic, and molecular evidence all suggest that the PDL may play a significant role in the treatment of this disease entity that is often difficult to manage and for which no standard treatment currently exists. Although the PDL has demonstrated efficacy and safety in a plethora of dermatologic research on cutaneous scar, only two papers to date demonstrate the use of the angiolytic laser for the treatment of vocal fold scar in humans[8,9]. Further research should be focused on determining the appropriate PDL, and KTP, laser parameters, technique and patient selection for optimization of vocal fold scar modulation.

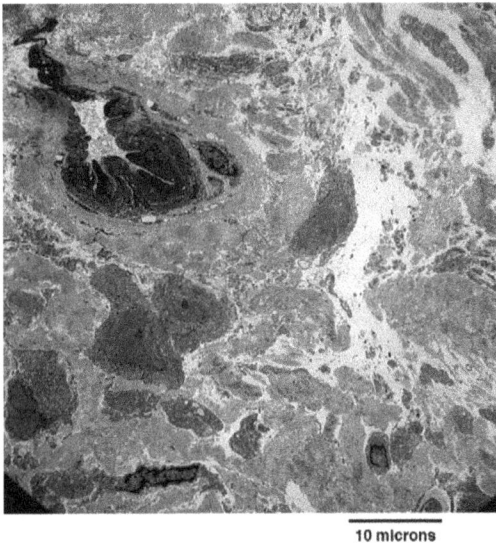

10 microns

Figure 9.5. Photocoagulation of a blood vessel within the SLP. This is the primary site of action for the PDL energy as it is absorbed by the oxyhemoglobin within the red blood cells. A proportion of the absorbed laser energy is liberated as heat from the vessel; this heat may be responsible for the cellular destruction that is observed within the epithelium[12].

References

1. Bredemeier HC. Laser accessory for surgical application. US Patent 3,659,613; issued 1972.
2. Rosen C, Simpson C. Principles of laser microsurgery. In: Rosen C, Simpson C, (Eds.). *Operative Techniques in Laryngology* Berlin, Heidelberg: Springer Verlag 2008.
3. Anderson R, Parrish J. Selective photothermolysis: precise microsurgery by selective absorption of pulsed radiation. *Science* 1983; 220:524–527.
4. Franco RA. In-office laryngeal surgery with the 585-nm pulsed dye laser. *Curr Opin Otolaryngol Head Neck Surg* 2007; 15:387–393

5. Zeitels SM, Burns JA. Office-based laryngeal laser surgery with the 532-nm pulsed-potassium-titanyl-phosphate laser. *Curr Opin Otolaryngol Head Neck Surg* 2007; 15:394–400.

6. Prufer N, Woo P, Altman K. Pulse dye and other laser treatment for vocal scar. *Curr Opin Otolaryngol Head Neck Surg* 2010; 18:492–497.

7. Alster T. Improvement of erythematous and hypertrophic scars by the 585-nm flashlamp-pumped pulsed dye laser. *Ann Plast Surg* 1994; 32:186–190.

8. Nouri K, Rivas M, Steven M, *et al.* Comparision of the effectiveness of the pulsed dye laser 585-nm versus 595-nm in the treatment of new surgical scars. *Lasers Med Sci* 2009; 24:801–810.

9. Hwang C, Lee H, Gyun J, *et al.* Use of pulsed dye laser in the treatment of sulcus vocalis. *Otolaryngol Head Neck Surg* 2013; 148:804–809.

10. Lin Y, Yamashita M, Zhang J, *et al.* Pulsed dye laser induced inflammatory response and extracellular matrix turnover in rat vocal folds and vocal fold fibroblasts. *Lasers Surg Med* 2009; 41:585–594.

11. Ayala C, Selig M, Faquin W, Franco R. Ultrastructural evaluation of 585-nm pulsed-dye laser-treated glottal dysplasia. *J Voice* 2007; 21:119–126.

12. Franco R, Zeitels S, Farinelli W, Anderson R. 585-nm pulsed dye laser treatment of glottal papillomatosis. *Ann Oto Rhino Laryngol* 2002; 111:486–492.

13. Mortensen M, Woo P, Ivey C, *et al.* The use of pulse dye laser in the treatment of vocal fold scar: a preliminary study. *Laryngoscope* 2008; 118:1884–1888.

14. Sheu M, Sridharan S, Paul B, *et al.* The utility of the potassium titanyl phosphate laser in modulating vocal fold scar in a rat model. *Laryngoscope* 2013; 123:2189–2194.

15. Asilian A, Darougheh A, Shariati F. New combination of triamcinolone, 5-fluorouracil, and pulsed-dye laser for treatment of keloid and hypertrophic scars. *Dermatol Surg* 2006; 32:907–915.

10

Tissue engineering

Shigeru Hirano

Tissue engineering approach for vocal fold scarring

The vocal fold has unique vibratory properties that are not seen in any other part of the body. These unique properties are supported by its histological architecture[1], and disruption of the normal architecture, such as in scarring, causes severe dysphonia that is difficult to treat.

Histological alterations within the superficial lamina propria (SLP) causes stiffened mucosa in the scarred vocal fold [2]. Histological analysis of human scarred vocal fold tissue after cordectomy indicates increased and disorganized collagen that forms thick bundles, decrease of elastic fibers, and reduction of hyaluronic acid (HA) in the SLP [3] (Figure 10.1). This histological alteration causes fibrosis of the mucosa which leads to reduced viscoelastic properties. Increase of fibronectin in scarred vocal folds is also thought to increase stiffness of the mucosa. Animal studies using vocal fold scar models have also revealed similar histological findings [4-6]. It is necessary to restore this altered structure in order to regenerate the vocal fold.

Based on the findings described above, regeneration of the vocal fold requires several elements, including cells and extracellular matrix (ECM). The most important part is to restore the normal distribution of ECM in the lamina propria, which requires modulation of the cell function within the vocal fold. The targets of a regenerative approach should include the cells in the vocal fold including fibroblasts, endothelial cells, epithelial cells, etc.

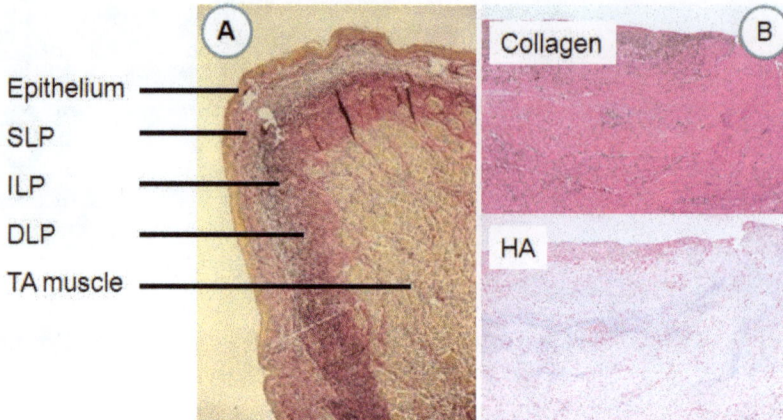

Figure 10.1. (A) Normal structure of human vocal fold presenting with layer structure of the lamina propria. (Cited from Reference #1, with permission). (B) Histology of human vocal fold scar. Note thick collagen deposition and loss of hyaluronic acid (HA). Cited from Reference #3, with permission.

Tissue engineering approaches involve cells, scaffolds, and regulatory factors (Figure 10.2). Among the most potent type of regulatory factors are growth factors which modulate cell function in terms of proliferation, migration, and ECM production. An appropriate combination of scaffold/cell/growth factor should be more effective at regenerating the vocal fold than any factor alone. The final goal of this tissue engineering strategy is to recover the normal histological structure of the vocal fold.

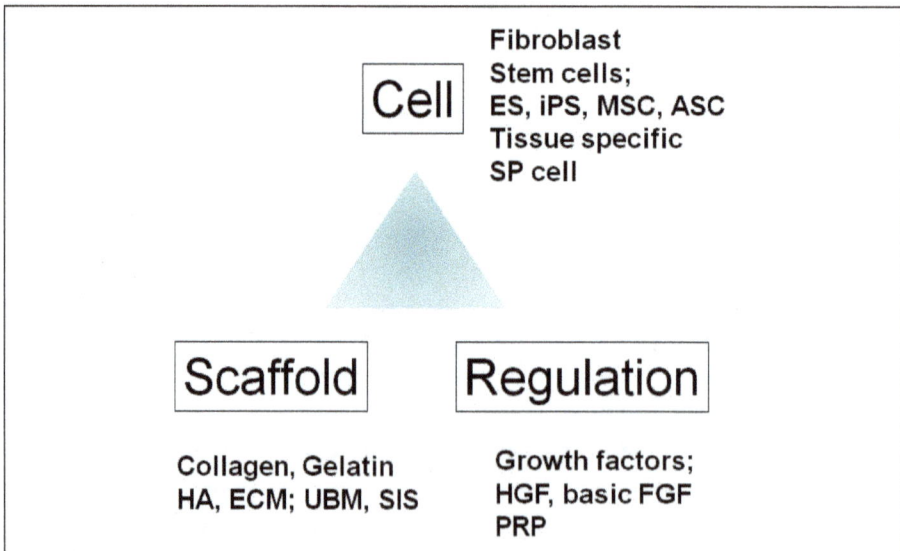

Figure 10.2. Concept and tools of tissue engineering approach.

Scaffolding

Scaffolding aims to regenerate tissue through implantation of regenerative scaffold into the target organ (Figure 10.3). Ideal regenerative scaffolds should be biocompatible and biodegradable. They should also possess characteristics which stimulate the influx of cells and growth factors from surrounding tissues. A favorable interaction between scaffold and cells and/or growth factors will lead to the formation of new, healthy tissue. The scaffold should be absorbed over time, but should remain for a certain period in order to complete the formation of new tissues. Several types of scaffolds have been studied for use in regeneration of the vocal fold, including collagen, gelatin, hyaluronic acid-based scaffolds, fascia, and decellularized bioscaffolds.

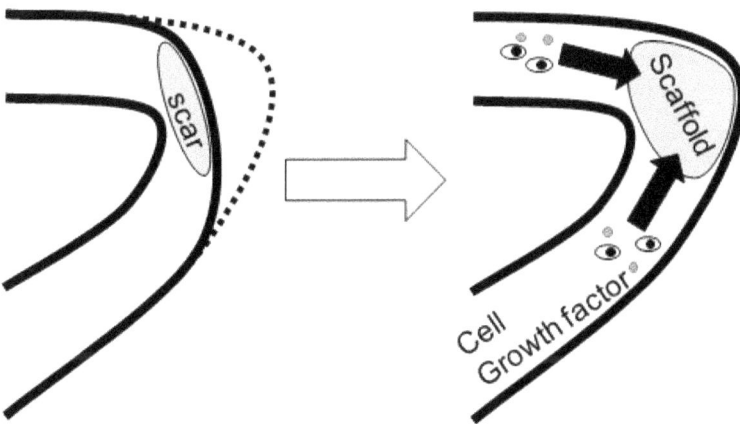

Figure 10.3. Concept of scaffolding surgery.

Collagen-gelatin material

Collagen or gelatin are relatively old materials, but are still useful as a scaffold for tissue regeneration. The feasibility of bovine-derived atelocollagen sponge (Terdermis®R, Terumo Co., Tokyo) was examined as a scaffold for vocal fold regeneration. To confirm biocompatibility of the scaffold, rat mesenchymal stem cells (MSCs) were cultured on the scaffold, and it was found that the cells survive, proliferate, and produce fibronectin.[7] A subsequent in vivo study[8] examined the effects of implanting the material into scarred vocal folds in a canine model. The results indicated that scarred canine vocal folds were softened and showed improvement of vibratory function. Histological analysis also showed recovery of hyaluronic acid (HA) in the lamina propria of the vocal fold. These effects were strengthened by combining the scaffold with MSCs.

Kishimoto *et al.* reported preliminary results on implant of this scaffold into scarred vocal folds or vocal fold sulcus in human patients[9] (Figure 10.4). The results showed gradual improvement of acoustic parameters of voice over six months to one year, although individual variation was noted. Scaffolding may be the most feasible method usable for human subjects.

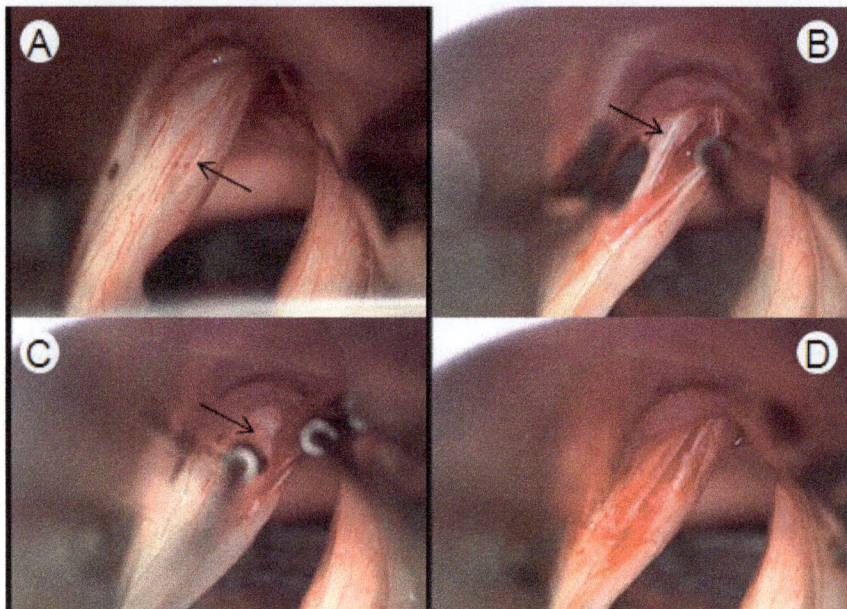

Figure 10.4. Regenerative surgery consisting of dissection of scar/sulcus using microflap technique (A-B), implant of regenerative material (C-D). Cited from Reference #60, with permission.

Gelatin is a solubilized form of collagen, and may also have a potential as a regenerative scaffold for the vocal fold. Zhang *et al.*[10] treated 12 patients with sulcus vocalis by implant of gelatin sponge coupled with fat injection. Improved maximum phonation time (MPT), shimmer, jitter, and noise ratio were reported at six months after the procedures. The effects of gelatin alone, however, are not clear because of the combined use of fat injection; however, gelatin is known to adhere to growth factors, and can act as a growth factor drug delivery system due to its unique characteristics, as will be described below.

Hyaluronic acid-based hydrogel

Hyaluronic acid (HA) has also received widespread attention as a candidate for regenerative scaffold for the vocal fold. HA is regarded as the key molecule for maintaining ideal viscoelasticity of the vocal fold mucosa. Boston group has developed an HA-based "microgel" as an injectable material for the vocal fold[11] and an in vitro study using fibroblast cultures showed low or no toxicity. Mechanical measurements taken with a torsional wave apparatus indicated that this HA-based microgel exhibited elastic moduli similar to the vocal fold lamina propria at frequencies close to the range of human phonation. This study suggested usefulness of the microgel for regeneration of the vocal fold lamina propria.

A Madison (Wisconsin) group has also developed a different type of HA hydrogels [12]. These chemically modified HA-gelatin hydrogels were implanted into the injured vocal folds of rabbits, and gene expression analysis of the treated vocal folds indicated up-regulated levels of mRNA for procollagen type I, fibronectin, TGF-beta1, fibromodulin, HA-Synthase 2, and hyaluronidase 2. The treated vocal folds also showed significantly improved tissue elasticity and viscosity.

One concern of the HA-based materials is that they are artificial forms of HA and they are not the native type of HA that naturally exists in the vocal fold. The characteristics of native HA have not been revealed. It is known that the biological behavior of HA depends on its molecular weight as Munoz-Pinto *et al.*[13] demonstrated that vocal fold fibroblasts cultured in HA hydrogels showed different gene expression according to the molecular weight of the HA. Thus, it will be important to explore the ideal molecular weight of HA.

Decellularized ECM ("Bioscaffold")

Decellularized ECM is a relatively new material and may have promising potential as a regenerative scaffold. Decellularization can be achieved by physical, chemical, or enzymatic processes[14]. Recent reports have demonstrated successful decellularization of whole organs including the heart, lung, kidney, liver, bowel, and skeletal muscle[15]. The technique allows production of complex 3D ECM bioscaffolds preserving the intrinsic vascular networks as well as ECM components. Recellularization is possible by perfusion of autologous stem cells. Xu *et al.*[16] developed an acellular xenogeneic ECM scaffold derived from bovine vocal fold lamina propria, and showed the biocompatibility of the scaffold with human vocal fold fibroblasts.

Badylak *et al.*[17] developed a porcine urinary bladder-derived ECM scaffold (UBM). UBM contains several growth factors as well as ECM components. Kitamura *et al.* have applied UBM to the defects of hemilaryngectomy using canine larynx, and confirmed simultaneous regeneration of the cartilage, muscle and the vocal fold mucosa[18] (Figure 10.5). Initial regeneration of the mucosa was observed quickly at two weeks after the implant. While the vibratory property of the mucosa varied by individual, the scaffold represents a promising material for laryngeal regeneration.

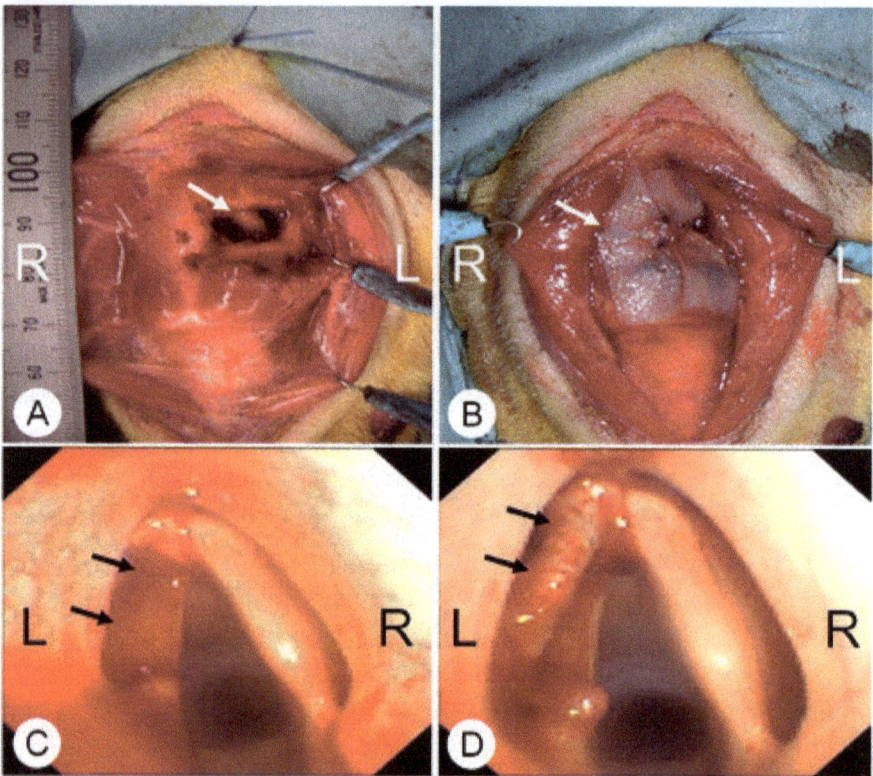

Figure 10.5. Regeneration of hemi-larynx using urinary bladder derived scaffold (UBM). (A) defect of hemi-laryngectomy of canine, (B) implant of UBM, (C) endoscopic findings after hemi-laryngectomy, (D) endoscopic findings after implant of UBM, (E) endoscopic findings 1 month after implant. Cited from Reference #18 with permission.

Small intestine submucosal scaffold (SIS) is another refined decelluralized scaffold that contains several types of ECM and growth factors including collagen, glycosaminoglycans, fibronectins, hyaluronic acids, basic fibroblast growth factor (bFGF), transforming growth factor-β (TGF-β), epidermal growth factor (EGF), vascular endothelial growth factor (VEGF). Choi *et al.* implanted SIS with bone marrow derived mesenchymal stem cell (MSC) into injured vocal folds of rabbits, and found recovery of histology with increased hyaluronic acid and controlled collage deposition[19].

These kinds of decellularized ECM scaffold may provide an ideal space for tissue regeneration because of the rich components including, not only ECM elements, but also growth factors and cytokines.

Cell therapy

Cell therapy is the main part and the most effective tool of tissue engineering. Cells can be delivered into the vocal fold with or without scaffolds. Once implanted, they proliferate, migrate, produce ECM proteins, and then lead to reformation of the histological architecture of the mucosa. Several types of cells have been studied as candidates for use in vocal fold regeneration, including mature and immature cells. Stem cells are expected to differentiate into different types of cells, and also to work in a paracrine way by producing several kinds of growth factors and cytokines.

Fibroblasts

The fibroblast is the main mature cell that exists in the vocal fold lamina propria, and there are some reports on use of fibroblasts for vocal fold scar in animal models. Hirano *et al.* attempted to implant vocal fold derived fibroblasts for the restoration of scarred canine vocal folds[20], but the results were disappointing because the treated vocal folds remained severely scarred, possibly because the control or function of implanted fibroblasts were not appropriate. A group at UCLA also conducted fibroblast injection into injured canine vocal folds[21] using autologous buccal mucosa fibroblasts, and the results were encouraging, showing improved mucosal wave of the vocal folds. The key question is how to control ECM production from the fibroblasts that are implanted into the vocal fold. To date, as the control of mature cells is not so easy, many researchers now focus more on immature cells, including several types of stem cells.

Bone marrow-derived mesenchymal stem cells (MSCs)

The bone marrow contains mesenchymal stem cells (MSC) as well as hematopoietic stem cells. MSCs are proven to be multipotent and to have ability to differentiate into several tissues including muscle, nerve, cartilage, tendon, fat, etc. It has also been shown that MSCs contribute to wound healing[22]. A population of MSCs circulates in the peripheral vessels and once tissue is damaged, the circulating MSCs are reported to migrate and home in to the injury site to repair the tissue.

Paracrine effects of MSCs are the other important function. MSCs produce several kinds of growth factors as well as ECM such as hepatocyte growth factor (HGF), vascular endothelial growth factor (VEGF), and collagen[23]. Ohno *et al.* demonstrated that MSCs have significantly higher levels of mRNA expression of hyaluronic acid synthase (HAS) and MMP-1 than vocal fold fibroblasts, which led to the hypothesis that implantation of MSCs would be effective for vocal fold regeneration in cases of vocal fold scar[24].

Injection of MSCs into injured tissue has shown promising results. It was reported that MSCs injected around wound sites stimulated enhanced re-epithelialization, cell growth, and angiogenesis with increased levels of VEGF and angiopoietin-1[25]. Another study also indicated that exogenous MSCs increased formulation of collagen matrix and stimulated angiogenesis during early stages of wound healing[26]. Kanemaru *et al.* treated injured canine vocal folds by means of implant of MSCs with collagen gel scaffold[27]. The results demonstrated better tissue recovery of the injured vocal folds treated by MSCs. The implanted MSCs were positive for mesenchymal stem cell markers, including CD29, CD44, CD49e, and Sca-1. Moreover, implanted MSCs in nude rat vocal folds expressed keratin and desmin, markers of epithelial tissue and muscle, respectively[28]. The implanted MSCs were proven to differentiate into different tissues such as the epithelium, muscle, and mesenchyme.

Hertegard *et al.* also treated scarred rabbit vocal folds by injection of human MSCs, and examined the effects on tissue property of the vocal fold[29] They confirmed that the injected MSCs persisted for four weeks in the vocal folds. The results showed lower viscosity and elastic moduli of the treated vocal folds as compared to untreated scarred vocal folds. Histological analysis indicated less deposition of collagen type I.

Ohno *et al.* performed a combined therapy of collagen scaffold and MSCs for the treatment of canine scarred vocal folds[8]. They found better regeneration of the vocal folds treated with the combination therapy than those treated with scaffold alone. Scaffolds can retain the cells for a longer period, which is considered to prolong the paracrine effects by the stem cells. Since MSCs are a source of autologous cells, clinical application is most feasible.

Adipose-derived mesenchymal stem cells (ASCs)

Fat tissue also includes mesenchymal stem cells called ASCs. ASCs have similar biological activity as MSCs including the multipotent ability to differentiate into several kinds of cells. Cultured ASCs have been shown to produce HGF, IGF, VEGF, and other cytokines, and are regarded suitable for vocal fold regeneration [30].

Lee *et al.* treated injured canine vocal folds by injection of ASCs, and found the presence of cells within the tissue after 6 months [31]. The treated vocal folds appeared to show better morphology. It was suggested that the retained ASCs may work in a paracrine manner for regeneration of the vocal fold. Xu *et al.* also reported the effects of ASC implantation for scarred vocal folds of rabbits [32]. The results demonstrated better regeneration of the vocal folds as compared to those treated with scaffold only.

There have been few comparative studies between MSCs and ASCs in terms of their effects on vocal fold regeneration, although the effects are thought to be similar. Recently, Hiwatashi *et al.* [33] completed a comparative study using MSCs or ASCs for restoration of rat vocal fold scarring. Two-month-old vocal fold scars in rats were treated by injection of MSCs or ASCs, and histological and genetic examination was performed 3 months after treatment. Results showed improved histological distribution of hyaluronic acid and collagen in both treatment groups. However, PCR results indicated significant up-regulation of hyaluronic acid synthase only in the ASC group. Gene expression levels of fibroblast growth factor and hepatocyte growth factor were significantly up-regulated in both treatment groups, although the expression of HGF was higher in ASC-treated vocal folds than in MSC-treated. These results suggest an enhanced regenerative potential of ASCs over MSCs; however, further investigation will be needed before any final conclusions can be made.

Tissue-specific stem cells

It is now well known that many tissues have their own specific stem cells which reside permanently in most organs. The tissue-specific stem cells have been identified in the skin, intestine, eye, brain, muscle, and others. They are located in so called "niches", which corresponds to the follicular bulge of the skin. However, the tissue specific stem cell of the vocal fold has not been identified. Yamashita *et al.* attempted to identify side population (SP) cells in the vocal fold mucosa using FACS combined with Hoechst staining, and found that SP cells comprised approximately 0.2% of the cells in the human vocal fold mucosa[34]. SP cells are thought to include abundant stem cells, and are located at the epithelium as well as the lamina propria of the vocal fold. These findings indicate the possible presence of tissue-specific stem cells in the vocal fold.

SP cells are also reported to contribute in wound healing and tissue regeneration. Expression of SP cells in the vocal fold was examined using injured rat vocal fold models[35]. The results showed that the SP cells accumulated in the injured site during the early phase of wound healing, within 1 week, and they rapidly disappeared. It was suggested that SP cells may contribute to wound healing or possible regeneration of injured vocal folds during the early stages of the wound healing.

SP cells are thought to include several immature cells other than pure tissue stem cells. Future research is needed to confirm the presence of the tissue stem cells within the vocal fold. Once identified, they should become one of the most promising cell source for treatment of vocal fold scar.

Embryonic stem (ES) cells / induced pluripotent stem (iPS) cells

ES cells are the origin of every cell and every organ in the body, and have the most effective potential to regenerate any organ. The effects of ES cell injection was examined using scarred rabbit vocal folds. The results demonstrated significantly improved viscoelasticity of the vocal fold mucosa when treated with ES cells[36]. The injected ES cells retained within the tissue for 1 month. Although ES cells are the most powerful item for regeneration of the vocal fold, there are several problems associated with their use, including ethical issues, immune reaction, and tumor formation. The research of ES cells has not progressed, at least in the field of laryngology.

The iPS cell was a breakthrough in stem cell technology and is regarded the most promising substitute for the use of ES cells. The iPS cells can be made from autologous tissues, which raises no ethical issues, or immune response. To date, unfortunately, there have been few studies about their use for the vocal fold. A significant concern surrounding iPS is the possibility of tumor formation. Imaizumi et al. first reported on the implantation of iPS cells into tracheal defects in rats, and obtained cartilage regeneration in 2 out of 5 rats, but they found teratoma formation in many cases[37]. Investigators in other fields are currently working to invent a technology to reduce the possibility of tumor formation. Recently. Imaizumi also reported successful differentiation of human iPS cells into vocal fold epithelial cells, which is encouraging for future iPS study[38].

Growth factor therapy

Growth factor therapy is another effective tool for tissue engineering. Exogenous growth factors stimulate cells inside the target organ, and modulate their function by changing their phenotype. Growth factor is expected to trigger a new process of wound healing or tissue regeneration, and thus even application of a growth factor in solution can have positive regenerative effects. It is also possible to develop more effective ways for delivery of growth factors to strengthen the effects.

Hepatocyte growth factor (HGF)

Hepatocyte growth factor (HGF) has strong anti-fibrotic activity, which makes it a promising candidate for treatment of vocal fold scar. HGF was first identified as a growth factor for hepatocytes, but subsequently it was revealed that HGF is produced and expressed in many organs and contributes to organogenesis, angiogenesis, and regeneration of several tissue types and organs[39].

Hirano et al. have confirmed that HGF is produced by vocal fold fibroblasts, and that the vocal folds express the HGF receptor, c-Met[40]. They also demonstrated that HGF stimulates production of hyaluronic acid (HA) and suppresses collagen synthesis by vocal fold fibroblasts, which are regarded as positive effects for the prevention or treatment of vocal fold scarring[41]. Krishna et al. reported increased production of HAS from rabbit vocal fold fibroblasts when HGF was applied[42]. Luo et al. reported that HGF stimulated production of HA and elastin

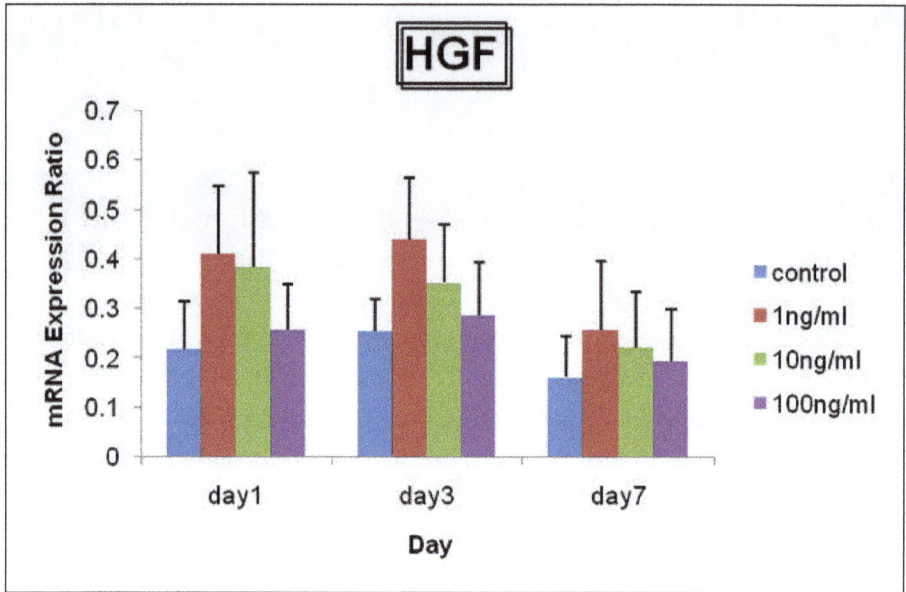

Figure 10.6. Autocrine effect of HGF. Endogenous HGF was up-regulated by administration of exogenous HGF to vocal fold fibroblast culture. Modified from Reference #44.

and suppressed collagen deposition in three dimensional cultures of fibroblasts in hydrogel[43]. Kishimoto *et al.* confirmed that exogenous HGF causes increased production of endogenous HGF from vocal fold cells, suggesting an autocrine loop for HGF signaling[44] (Figure 10.6).

In vivo studies using rabbits and dogs showed significant regenerative effects of HGF for the prevention and treatment of scarred vocal folds. In a rabbit study, HGF was administered just after stripping the vocal folds, and the results showed better wound healing, with regeneration of the lamina propria in the treated vocal folds[45]. Viscosity and stiffness of the vocal folds were also significantly improved by the treatment of HGF compared to non-treated, scarred vocal folds. In a canine study, month-old scars of the vocal fold were injected with HGF, and the results indicated better tissue properties and improved histological architecture of the vocal fold mucosa, with restored levels of HA and abundant, well organized collagen at 6 months after the treatment[46] (Figure 10.7).

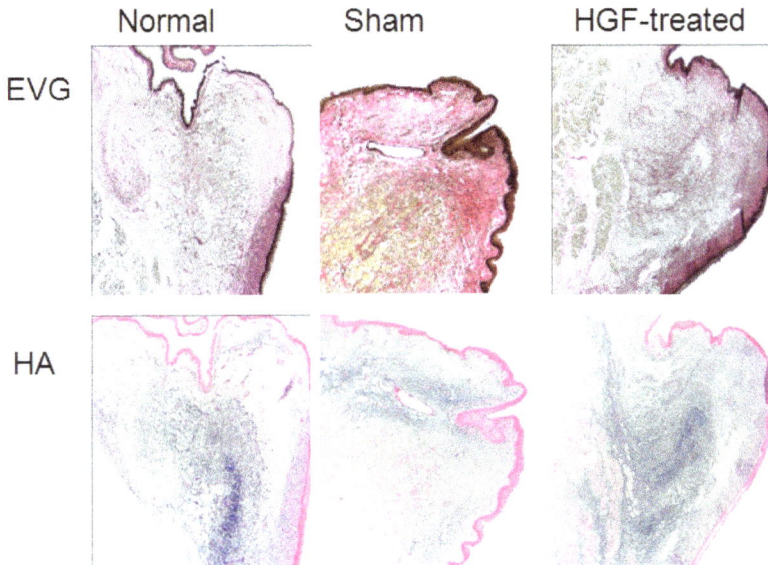

Figure 10.7. Effects of HGF injection into scarred canine vocal folds. The vocal fold structure was well restored by HGF injection. EVG: elastic-von-Gieson stain, HA: hyaluronic acid. Cited from Reference #46 with permission.

A novel drug delivery system for HGF was developed using gelatin hydrogel, which enabled the controlled-released of HGF within the tissue over a 2 week period. This drug delivery system has proven to be useful even for the treatment of chronic scarring of the vocal fold (6 months scar) in another canine model[47].

It has also been proven that HGF is effective for the treatment of aged vocal fold atrophy. Ohno *et al*. locally applied HGF to aged rat vocal folds and confirmed up-regulation of mRNA expression of HAS and MMP in the treated vocal folds, with improved histology of the aged vocal folds, indicating increased HA and decreased collagen[48]. Suehiro *et al*. examined the optimal dose of HGF for the treatment of aged vocal fold atrophy in rats, and found that the most favorable biochemical effects of HGF occurred at a concentration of 100 ng/10 µL, based on the ability to up-regulate the expression of HAS-2 and MMP-9 mRNA, and to down-regulate the expression of collagen type I[49].

As described above, HGF is a promising tool for the regenerative treatment of vocal fold scarring, sulcus, and atrophy, but unfortunately there is presently no commercial product available for human use. Recently, 5 amino acid-deleted type HGF (dHGF) was developed in good manufacturing practices (GMP) which is compatible for use in humans[50]. This form of dHGF has been shown to have similar biological activity to full-length HGF. A comparative study was conducted to clarify the difference of effects on vocal fold scar between both HGFs using a canine model, and the results confirmed that both forms of HGF have similar regenerative effects on the vocal fold in terms of vibratory function and histological aspects[51]. A clinical trial is expected using the GMP-compatible HGF product in the future.

Basic fibroblast growth factor (bFGF)

Basic FGF is another regenerative medicine candidate for vocal fold scar. It is a stimulant of fibroblasts and induces cell migration and proliferation. It also contributes in stimulating angiogenesis and epithelialization. Several in vitro studies have demonstrated that bFGF stimulates HA synthesis and suppresses collagen gene expression[52,53]. It has also been reported that bFGF stimulates HA production from aged rat vocal fold fibroblasts. Subsequent in vivo study has confirmed its regenerative effects by injecting bFGF into aged rat vocal folds[54,55]. Histological examination indicated that bFGF-treated vocal folds showed recovery of HA distribution in the lamina propria with reduced collagen deposition (Figure 10.8). Ohno et al. further examined these effects at the genetic level using PCR[56], and then found that bFGF up-regulated hyaluronic acid synthase (HAS) 2 and 3, MMP2 in aged rat vocal folds. Based on this basic research, a clinical trial was performed for human subjects with aged vocal fold atrophy. The subjects were treated with local injection of the bFGF product Fibrast® (Kaken Co., Tokyo). The first case was reported in 2008 with excellent results indicating improved vibratory properties with better voice after administration of bFGF[57] (Figure 10.9). Ten cases were finally recruited and analyzed, and the data showed improved phonatory function including MPT, jitter, shimmer, and noise parameters. Mucosal wave amplitude of the vocal folds was also significantly improved in a period of up to 1 year after treatment[58].

Basic FGF was then applied to vocal fold scar. Suehiro et al. attempted to treat vocal fold scarring with bFGF in a canine study, in which repeated injection of bFGF solution caused restoration of scarred vocal folds in terms of mucosal vibration and histological findings[59]. In the clinical setting, bFGF has been applied to human cases of vocal fold scar or sulcus by means of injection of bFGF solution or regenerative surgery (Figure 10.4). Regenerative surgery consists of elevation of a microflap, dissection of scar in the lamina propria, and implantation of gelatin scaffold with bFGF[60]. The results showed significant improvement in MPT, GRBAS scale, and voice handicap index -10, with improved vibratory function (Figure 10.10). Although improvement of acoustic

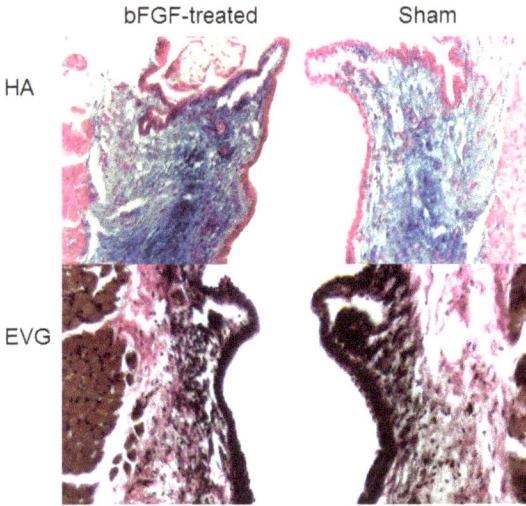

Figure 10.8. Effects of injection of basic FGF into aged rat vocal folds. Basic FGF significantly increased hyaluronic acid deposition. Cited from Reference #55 with permission.

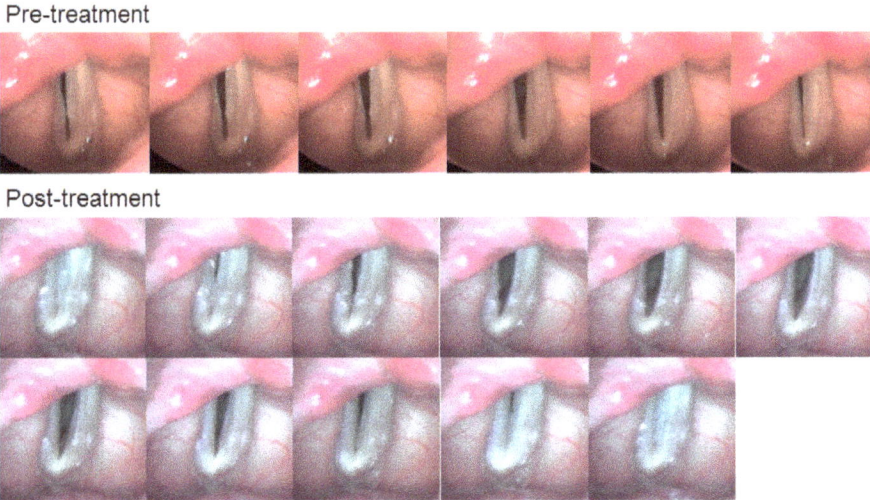

Figure 10.9. Basic FGF injection into human aged atrophy of the vocal fold. Pre-treatment image indicates small amplitude of mucosal wave with glottis gap, while post-treatment images show improved vibratory amplitude with complete glottis closure.

Pre-treatment

Post-treatment

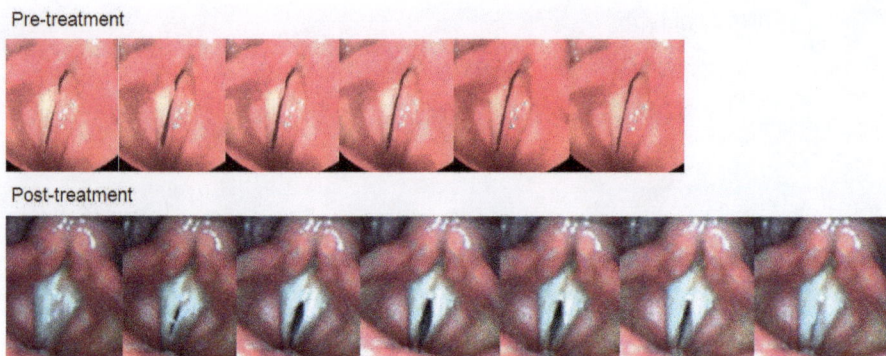

Figure 10.10. Basic FGF treatment for human vocal fold scar. Pre-treatment: both vocal folds rarely move. Post-treatment: Both vocal folds vibrates well with complete glottis closure.

parameters varied across cases, bFGF has proven to have a therapeutic effects for vocal fold scar.

In conclusion, the therapeutic effects of both HGF and bFGF have been confirmed for either scarred or atrophied vocal folds.

Future directions

Regeneration of the vocal fold remains challenging because the vocal fold has sophisticated layered structure with vibratory properties, which are difficult to restore. Growth factors, with or without scaffold, are feasible and effective for clinical application. One of the main issues may be how to strengthen the effects and improve consistency across individual cases. A novel drug delivery system (DDS) should be developed to resolve this aspect. Gelatin may be the best scaffold for growth factors as a DDS carrier now, but more optimal materials should be explored. Another issue is the determination of the most suitable growth factor for vocal fold regeneration. To date, bFGF and HGF have proven to be promising factors, but it is not yet known which is better, or the advantages and disadvantages of each growth factor compared to the other. Recently plasma-rich platelet (PRP) has received more attention for regeneration of several tissues and organs because PRP includes several kinds of growth factors and cytokines ("cocktail of cytokine"). A comparative study among each material is thus warranted in the future.

Generally, cell therapy is the strongest tool for regeneration of any organs. Several cell sources are available including MSCs, ASCs, or even iPS cells, although it is also not known which is best, or what advantage each cell source has over the other. Clinical trials are needed to confirm the safety and efficacy of each cell source. Tumor formation must be excluded.

Decellularized ECM scaffolding may have great potential for regenerating not only the vocal fold but also whole larynx. This strategy may make it possible to regenerate the larynx after total laryngectomy. Ideal methods to decellularize the larynx should be explored preserving important architecture such as cartilage, muscular structure, mucosa, vessels and nerves.

Given that the larynx is the most important organ for vocal communication output, it is essential to continuously develop regenerative medicine for the larynx.

References

1. Hirano M. Phonosurgery. Basic and clinical investigations. *Otologia (Fukuoka)* 1975; 21:239–440.
2. Hirano S. Current treatment of vocal fold scarring. *Curr Opin Otolaryngol Head Neck Surg* 2005; 13(3):143–147.
3. Hirano S, Minamiguchi S, Yamashita M, *et al.* Histologic characterization of human scarred vocal folds. *J Voice* 2009; 23(4):399–407.
4. Rousseau B, Hirano S, Scheidt TD, *et al.* Characterization of vocal fold scarring in a canine model. *Laryngoscope* 2003; 113:620–627.
5. Hirano S, Bless DM, Rousseau B, *et al.* Fibronectin and adhesion molecules on canine scarred vocal folds. *Laryngoscope* 2003; 113:966–972.
6. Thibeault SL, Bless DM, Gray SD. Interstitial protein alterations in rabbit vocal fold with scar. *J Voice* 2003; 17:377–383.
7. Ohno S, Hirano S, Tateya I, *et al.* Atelocollagen sponge as a stem cell implantation scaffold for the treatment of scarred vocal fold. *Ann Otol Rhinol Laryngol* 2009; 118:805–810.
8. Ohno S, Hirano S, Kanemaru S, *et al.* Implantation of an atelocollagen sponge with autologous bone marrow derived mesenchymal stromal cells for treatment of vocal fold scarring in a canine model. *Ann Otol Rhinol Laryngol* 2011; 120:401–408.
9. Kishimoto Y, Hirano S, Kojima T, *et al.* Implant of atelocollagen sheet for the treatment of vocal fold scarring and sulcus vocalis. *Ann Otol Rhinol Larngol* 2009; 118:613–620.
10. Zhang F, Sprecher AJ, Wei C, *et al.* Implantation of gelatin sponge combined with injectin of autologous fat for sulcus vocalis. *Otolaryngol Head Neck Surg* 2010; 143:198–203.

11. Jia X, Yeo Y, Clifton RJ, *et al*. Hyaluronic acid-based microgels and microgel networks for vocal fold regeneration. *Biomacromolecules* 2006; 7(12):3336–3344.
12. Duflo S, Thibeault SL, Li W, *et al*. Vocal fold tissue repair in vivo using a synthetic extracellular matrix. *Tissue Eng* 2006; 12(8):2171–2180.
13. Munoz-Pinto DJ, Jimenez-Vergara AC, Gelves LM, *et al*. Probing vocal fold fibroblast response to hyalurona in 3D contexts. *Biotechnol Bioeng* 2009; 104:821–31.
14. Gilbert TW, Sellaro Tl, Badylak SF. Decellularization of organs and tissues. *Biomaterial* 2006; 27:3675–3683.
15. He M, Callanan A. Comparison of methods for whole-organ decellularization in tissue engineering of bioartificial organs. *Tissue Eng* Part B 2013; 19:1–11.
16. Xu CC, Chan RW, Tirunagari N. A biodegradable, acellular xenogeneic scaffold for regeneration of the vocal fold lamina propria. *Tissue Eng* 2007; 13:551–566.
17. Badylak SF, Freytes DO, Gilbert TW: Extracellular matrix as a biologic scaffold material: structure and function. *Acta Biomaterialia* 2009; 5(1): 1–13.
18. Kitamura M, Hirano S, Kanemaru S, *et al*. Glottic regeneration with tissue engineering technique using acellular extracellular matrix scaffold in canine model. *J Tissue Eng Rregen Med* 2014 Jan 8; doi: 10.1002/term.1855
19. Choi JW, Park JK, Chang JW, *et al*. Small intestine submucosa and mesenchymal stem cells composite gel for scarless vocal fold regeneration. *Biomaterials* 2014; 35(18):4911–4918.
20. Hirano S, Bless DM, Nagai H, *et al*. Growth factor therapy for vocal fold scarring in canine model. *Ann Otol Rhinol Laryngol* 2004;113:777–785.
21. Chhetri DK, Head C, Revazova E, *et al*. Lamina propria replacement therapy with cultured autologous fibroblasts for vocal fold scars. *Otolaryngol Head Neck Surg* 2004; 131:864–870.
22. Le Blanc K. Mesenchymal stromal cells: Tissue repair and immune modulation *Cytotherapy* 2006; 8:559–61.
23. Han SK, *et al*. Potential of human bone marrow stromal cells to accelerate wound healing in vitro *Ann Plast Surg* 2005; 55:414–419Ohno T, Hirano S, Kanemaru S, *et al*. Expression of extracellular matrix proteins in the vocal folds and bone marrow derived stromal cells of rats. *Eur Arch Otorhinolaryngol* 2008; 265:669–674.
24. Wu Y, Chen L, Scott PG, *et al*. Mesenchymal stem cells enhance wound healing through differentiation and angiogenesis. *Stem Cells* 2007 Oct; 25(10):2648–2659.
25. Ichioka S, Kouraba S, Sekiya N, *et al*. Bone marrow impregnated collagen matrix for wound healing: experimental evaluation in a microcirculatory model of angiogenesis and clinical experience. *Br J Plast Surg* 2005; 58:1124–30.
26. Kanemaru S, Nakamura T, Omori K, *et al*. Regeneration of the vocal fold using autologous mesenchymal stem cells. *Ann Otol Rhinol Laryngol* 2003; 112:915–920.
27. Kanemaru S, Nakamura T, Yamashita M, *et al*. Destiny of autologous bone marrow-derived stromal cells implanted in the vocal fold. *Ann Otol Rhinol Laryngol* 2005; 114(12):907–912.

28. Hertegard S, Cedervall J, Svensson B, *et al.* Viscoelastic and histologic properties in scarred rabbit vocal folds after mesenchymal stem cell injection. *Laryngoscope* 2006; 116(7):1248–1254.

29. Yoshida A, Kitajiri S, Nakagawa T, *et al.* Adipose tissue-derived stromal cells protect hair cells from aminoglycoside. *Laryngoscope* 2011; 121(6):1281–1286.

30. Lee BJ, Wang SG, Lee JC, *et al.* The prevention of vocal fold scarring using autologous adipose tissue-derived stromal cells. *Cells Tissues Organs* 2006; 184(3–4):198–204.

31. Xu W, Hu R, Fan E, *et al.* Adipose derived mesenchymal stem cells in collagen hyaluronic acid gel composite scaffolds for vocal fold regeneration. *Ann Otol Rhinol Laryngol* 2011; 120:123–130.

32. Hiwatashi N, Hirano S, Mizuta M, *et al.* Adipose-derived stem cells versus bone marrow-derived stem cells for vocal fold regeneration. *Laryngoscope* 2014; 124(12):E461–E469.

33. Yamashita M, Hirano S, Kanemaru S, *et al.* Side population cells in the human vocal fold. *Ann Otol Rhinol Laryngol* 2007; 116:853–857.

34. Gugatschka M, Kojima T, Ohno S, *et al.* Recruitment patterns of side population cells during wound healing in rat vocal folds. *Laryngoscope* 2011; 121:1662–1667.

35. Cedervall J, Ahrlund-Richter L, Svensson B, *et al.* Injection of embryonic stem cells into scarred rabbit vocal folds enhances healing and improves viscoelasticity: short-term results *Laryngoscope* 2007; 117(11):2075–2081.

36 Imaizumi M, Nomoto Y, Sugino T, *et al.* Potential of induced pluripotent stem cells for the regeneration of the tracheal wall. *Ann Otol Rhinol Laryngol* 2010; 119(10):697–703.

37. Imaizumi M, Sato Y, Yang DT, *et al.* In vitro epithelial differentiation of human induced pluripotent stem cells for vocal fold tissue engineering. *Ann Otol Rhinol Laryngol* 2014; 122:737–747.

38. Matsumoto K, Nakamura T. Hepatocyte growth factor (HGF) as a tissue organizer for organogenesis and regeneration. *Biochem Biophys Res Commun* 1997; 239:639–644.

39. Hirano S, Thibeault S, Bless DM, *et al.* Hepatocyte growth factor and its receptor c-met in rat and rabbit vocal folds. *Ann Otol Rhinol Laryngol* 2002; 111:661–666.

40. Hirano S, Bless D, Heisey D, *et al.* Roles of hepatocyte growth factor and transforming growth factor beta1 in production of extracellular matrix by canine vocal fold fibroblasts *Laryngoscope* 2003; 113:144–148.

41. Krishna P, Rosen CA, Branski RC, *et al.* Primed fibroblasts and exogenous decorin: Potential treatments for subacute vocal fold scar. *Otolaryngol Head Neck Surg* 2006; 135(6):937–945.

42. Luo Y, Kobler JB, Zeitels SM, *et al.* Effects of growth factors on extracellular matrix production by vocal fold fibroblasts in 3-dimensional culture. *Tissue Eng* 2006; 12(12):3365–3374.

43. Kishimoto Y, Hirano S, Suehiro A, *et al.* Effect of exogenous hepatocyte growth factor on vocal fold fibroblasts. *Ann Otol Rhinol Laryngol* 2009; 118:606–611.

44. Hirano S, Bless DM, Rousseau B, *et al.* Prevention of vocal fold scarring by topical injection of hepatocyte growth factor in rabbit model. *Laryngoscope* 2004; 114:548–556.

45. Hirano S, Bless DM, Nagai H, *et al.* growth factor therapy for vocal fold scarring in canine model. *Ann Otol Rhinol Laryngol* 2004; 113:777–785.

46. Kishimoto Y, Hirano S, Kitani Y, *et al.* Chronic vocal fold scar restoration with hepatocyte growth factor. *Laryngoscope* 2010; 120:108–113.

47. Ohno T, Yoo MJ, Swanson E, *et al.* Regeneration of aged rat vocal folds using hepatocyte growth factor therapy. *Laryngoscope* 2009; 119:1424–1430.

48. Suehiro A, Wright H, Rousseau B. Optimal concentration of hepatocyte growth factor for treatment of the aged rat vocal fold. *Laryngoscope* 2011; 121:1726–1734.

49. Shima N, Tsuda E, Goto M, *et al.* Hepatocyte growth factor and its variant with a deletion of five amino acids are distinguishable in their biological activity and tertiary structure. *Biochem Biophys Res Commun* 1994; 200:808–815.

50. Mizuta M, Hirano S, Ohno S, *et al.* Restoration of scarred vocal folds using 5 amino acid-deleted type hepatocyte growth factor. *Laryngoscope* 2014; 124(3):E81–E86.

51. Heldin P, Laurent TC, Heldin CH. Effect of growth factors on hyaluronan synthesis in cultured human fibroblasts. *Biochem J* 1989; 258:919–922.

52. Hong HH, Trackman PC. Cytokine regulation of gingival fibroblast lysyl oxidase, collagen, and elastin. *J Periodontol* 2002; 73:145–152.

53. Hirano S, Bless DM, Muñoz del Río A, *et al.* therapeutic potential of growth factors for aging voice. *Laryngoscope* 2004; 114:2161–2167.

54. Hirano S, Nagai H, Tateya I, *et al.* Regeneration of aged vocal folds with basic fibroblast growth factor in a rat model: A preliminary report. *Ann Otol Rhinol Laryngol* 2005; 114:304–308.

55. Ohno T, Jin Yoo M, Swanson ER, *et al.* Regenerative effects of basic growth factor on extracellular matrix production in aged rat vocal folds. *Ann Otol Rhinol Laryngol* 2009; 118:559–564.

56. Hirano S, Kishimoto Y, Suehiro A, *et al.* Regeneration of aged vocal fold: First human case treated with fibroblast growth factor. *Laryngoscope* 2008; 118:2254–2259.

57. Hirano S, Tateya I, Kishimoto Y, *et al.* Clinical trial of regeneration of aged vocal folds with growth factor therapy. *Laryngoscope* 2012; 122:327–331.

58. Suehiro A, Hirano S, Kishimoto Y, *et al.* Treatment of acute vocal fold scar with local injection of basic fibroblast growth factor: A canine study. *Acta Otolaryngol* 2010; 130(7):844–850.

59. Hirano S, Mizuta M, Kaneko M, *et al.* Regenerative phonosurgical treatments for vocal fold scar and sulcus with basic fibroblast growth factor. *Laryngoscope* 2013; 123(11):2749–2755.

Index

phase space reconstruction, acoustic
analysis, 30
phonation quality. *see* dysphonia
phonation quotient (PQ), aerodynamic
measures, 31
phonation threshold pressure (PTP),
aerodynamic measures, 31
Phonatory Aerodynamic System (PAS),
43
phonetogram, 29
phonotrauma
causes of scarring, **19**, 19–20, 118
sulcus vocalis, 96
voice therapy, 41
photoangiolytic glottoplasty, sulcus
vocalis, 102
photoangiolytic lasers, subepithelial
infusion, 76
physical examination, diagnostic, 25–27
pig models
tissue engineering, 146
vocal fold rehabilitation, 14
wound healing, 10
pitch glides, voice therapy, 48, 49, 50
plasma-rich platelet (PRP) tissue
engineering, *142*, 156
polyps, 20, 97
posterior glottic stenosis, medical
management, 60
posterior transverse laser cordotomy,
medical management, 58
post-operative care
laryngeal resurfacing, 130–131
sulcus vocalis, 113
voice therapy, 51–52
post-operative dysphonia, 21
post-processed iScan, 34
posture, voice therapy, 45, 46
potassium titanyl phosphate. *see* KTP
laser treatment
PQ (phonation quotient), aerodynamic
measures, 31
prednisolone, **57**
prednisone, **57**
pre-processed narrow band imaging, 34
prevalence, voice difficulties, 3, 95–96,
98

prevention of vocal problems, 13–15. *see
also* voice therapy
Prolaryn Gel®, 65, **77**, *78*, **78**, 110
Prolaryn Plus®, 65, 68, *68*, 77, **77**, *78*, **78**,
110
proliferation, wound healing stages, 6, 7,
55
prophylactic medical management, 56, 58
protein synthesis, 4, 5, **10**, *55*, 58
proteoglycans, 8, 66
PRP (plasma-rich platelets), *142*, 156
PTP (phonation threshold pressure),
aerodynamic measures, 31
pulmonary function tests, aerodynamic
measures, 30–31
pulsed dye laser. *see* PDL

rabbit models
growth factor therapy, 152
medical management, 56, 58
molecular level changes, 13
tissue engineering, 147, 148
viscoelasticity in vocal fold scar, 11–13
wound healing, 6, 9, 10
Radiesse Voice® calcium hydroxylapatite,
68
radiotherapy, causes of scarring, 21
rat models
growth factor therapy, 154, *155*
pulsed dye laser treatment, 137
tissue engineering, 143, 149
wound healing, 6, 10
reconstructions, laryngeal resurfacing,
119, 121–123, *125–129*
recovery time frames. *see* time frames for
healing/recovery
recurrent respiratory papillomatosis,
causes of scarring, 21
reflux disease. *see* laryngopharyngeal
reflux
regularity, physical examination, 27
Reinke's edema, 20
Reinke's space, 7, 90–91, 103, 104
relaxation, voice therapy, 45–46, 48. *see
also* muscle tension
remodeling
scar formation, *55*

About the Editors

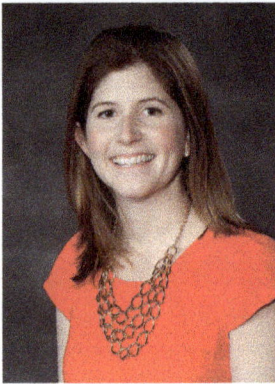

Jaime Eaglin Moore, M.D. is an otolaryngologist and laryngologist. Dr. Moore is board certified by the American Board of Otolaryngology. Dr. Moore received her Doctor of Medicine degree from Eastern Virginia Medical School, and she completed a residency in Otolaryngology – Head and Neck Surgery at Virginia Commonwealth University in Richmond, Virginia. She was a fellow in laryngology and care of the professional voice at the American Institute for Voice and Ear Research. Author of numerous publications and on the editorial board for the *Ear, Nose and Throat Journal* and the *Journal of Voice*, Dr. Moore is Assistant Professor Otolaryngology – Head and Neck Surgery and an Adjunct Professor in the Department of Music at Virginia Commonwealth University.

Mary J. Hawkshaw, B.S.N., R.N., CORLN is Professor in the Department of Otolaryngology – Head and Neck Surgery at Drexel University College of Medicine. She has been associated with Dr. Robert Sataloff, Philadelphia Ear, Nose & Throat Associates and the American Institute for Voice & Ear Research (AIVER) since 1986. Ms. Hawkshaw graduated from Shadyside Hospital School of Nursing in Pittsburgh, Pennsylvania and received a Bachelor of Science degree in Nursing from Thomas Jefferson University in Philadelphia.

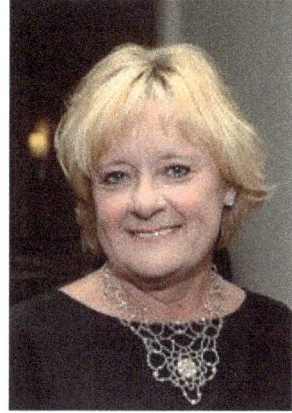

In addition to her specialized clinical activities, she has been involved extensively in research and teaching. She mentors medical students, residents, and laryngology fellows, and has been involved in teaching research, writing and editing for nearly three decades. In collaboration with Dr. Sataloff, she has co-authored more than 170 articles, 70 book chapters, and 10 textbooks. A member of the Editorial Boards of the *Journal of Voice* and *Ear, Nose and Throat Journal*, she has served as Secretary/Treasurer of AIVER since 1988 and was named Executive Director January 2000. She has served on the Board of Directors of the Voice Foundation since 1990. Ms. Hawkshaw has been an active member of the Society of Otorhinolaryngology and Head-Neck Nurses since 1998. She is recognized nationally and internationally for her extensive contributions to care of the professional voice.

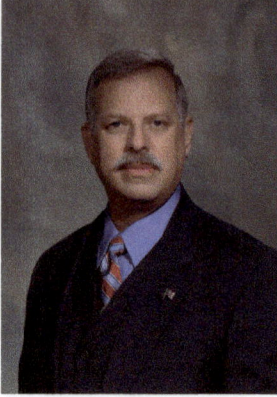

Robert T. Sataloff, M.D., D.M.A., F.A.C.S. is Professor and Chairman, Department of Otolaryngology-Head and Neck Surgery and Senior Associate Dean for Clinical Academic Specialties, Drexel University College of Medicine. He is also Adjunct Professor in the departments of Otolaryngology – Head and Neck Surgery at Thomas Jefferson University, the University of Pennsylvania, and Temple University; and on the faculty of the Academy of Vocal Arts. Dr. Sataloff is also a professional singer and singing teacher, and he served as Conductor of the Thomas Jefferson University Choir over a period of nearly four decades. He holds an undergraduate degree from Haverford College in Music Theory and Composition, graduated from Jefferson Medical College, Thomas Jefferson University, received a Doctor of Musical Arts in Voice Performance from Combs College of Music; and he completed his Residency in Otolaryngology – Head and Neck Surgery and a Fellowship in Otology, Neurotology and Skull Base Surgery at the University of Michigan. Dr. Sataloff is Chairman of the Boards of Directors of the Voice Foundation and of the American Institute for Voice and Ear Research. He has also served as Chairman of the Board of Governors of Graduate Hospital; President of the American Laryngological Association, the International Association of Phonosurgery, and the Pennsylvania Academy of Otolaryngology – Head and Neck Surgery; and in numerous other leadership positions. Dr. Sataloff is Editor-in-Chief of the *Journal of Voice*, Editor-in-Chief of *Ear, Nose and Throat Journal*, Editor-in-Chief of the *Journal of Case Reports in Medicine*, Associate Editor of the *Journal of Singing*, and on the editorial boards of numerous otolaryngology journals. He has written over 1,000 publications, including 59 books. His medical practice is limited to care of the professional voice and to otology/neurotology/skull base surgery.

www.ingramcontent.com/pod-product-compliance
Lightning Source LLC
Chambersburg PA
CBHW050106220326
41598CB00043B/7399